Tackling chronic disease in Europe

Strategies, interventions and challenges

Reinhard Busse

Miriam Blümel

David Scheller-Kreinsen

Annette Zentner

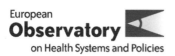

European
Observatory
on Health Systems and Policies

Keywords:

CHRONIC DISEASE – prevention and control – economics
COST OF ILLNESS
COST-BENEFIT ANALYSIS
STRATEGIC PLANNING
DELIVERY OF HEALTH CARE, INTEGRATED
EUROPE

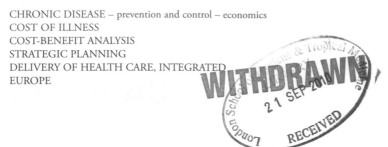

ISBN 9789289041928

Printed in the United Kingdom by The Cromwell Press Group

Contents

Acknowledgements   vii

List of tables, figures and boxes   ix

List of abbreviations   xi

About the authors   xiii

Chapter 1 Introduction   1

Part I: Burden of chronic disease

Chapter 2 Deaths and burden of chronic disease in Europe   9

      2.1 Current status   9

      2.2 Predictions   17

Chapter 3 Economic consequences of chronic disease   19

      3.1 The microeconomic perspective   19

      3.2 The macroeconomic perspective   24

Part II: Strategies for tackling chronic disease

Chapter 4 Strategies against chronic disease: what is being done?   27

      4.1 Prevention and early detection   27

      4.2 New provider qualifications and settings   31

      4.3 Coordinating care for individual chronic diseases: DMPs   34

      4.4 Managing care across chronic diseases: integrated care models   36

Chapter 5 Effectiveness of strategies against chronic disease   39

          5.1 Prevention and early detection   39

          5.2 New provider qualifications and settings   40

          5.3 Coordinating care for individual chronic diseases: DMPs 41

          5.4 Managing care across chronic diseases: integrated care models 45

Chapter 6 Cost–effectiveness of strategies against chronic disease   49

          6.1 Prevention and early detection   49

          6.2 New provider qualifications and settings   51

          6.3 Coordinating care for individual chronic diseases: DMPs 51

          6.4 Managing care across chronic diseases: integrated care models 52

Part III: Challenges of chronic disease management

Chapter 7 Tackling the challenges of chronic disease in Europe   55

          7.1 New pharmaceuticals and medical devices   55

          7.2 Financial incentives   59

          7.3 Improving coordination   67

          7.4 Information and communication technology   75

          7.5 Evaluation culture   79

Chapter 8 Conclusions   85

          References   91

Acknowledgements

The authors have built on work undertaken for the second report of the "Initiative for Sustainable Healthcare Financing in Europe", entitled *Securing Europe's Healthcare Future: Chronic Disease Management and Health Technology Assessment (2009)*, which was made possible by financial assistance from Pfizer Inc, and was endorsed by the Czech Presidency of the European Union and the Czech Ministry of Health. This book derives from that work and is developed from it.

The views expressed in this work are solely those of the authors and do not necessarily represent the views and policies of the organizations to which they belong or of those organizations that facilitated or funded the work.

The authors are extremely thankful for the comments and insights by the members of the steering committee for the Initiative for Sustainable Healthcare Financing in Europe: Pat Cox, Claude Hemmer, Elias Mossialos, Stephen Wright, Fabienne Bartoli, Panos Kanavos, Ulf Persson, Jack Watters and Jacques de Tournemire.

The authors would also like to thank their valued colleagues, Marilyn Clark and Ewout van Ginneken, who contributed formally and informally to the realization of the project.

List of tables, figures and boxes

Tables

Table 2.1   Disease burden and deaths from noncommunicable   10
diseases in the WHO European Region by cause (2005)

Table 2.2   Deaths and burden of disease attributable to common risk   12
factors, in absolute numbers and percentages of all deaths/
DALYs, by contribution to worldwide deaths (2001)

Table 3.1   Impact of chronic diseases and conditions and risk   20–21
factors on labour supply, selected examples

Table 3.2   Impact of chronic diseases and conditions and risk   21–23
factors on wages, earnings or incomes, selected examples

Table 4.1   Population goals for nutrients and features of lifestyle   29
consistent with the prevention of major public health
problems in Europe

Table 4.2   DMP participants in Germany according to indication   35
(2008)

Table 5.1   Effects of antismoking measures on smoker prevalence   40

Table 5.2   Summary of evidence for various disease management   43
programme outcomes, by disease

Table 5.3   Findings from studies of large-scale, population-based   44
disease management programmes

Table 5.4   Summary of evidence on effectiveness of CCM   46
components

Table 6.1   Cost per QALY saved by interventions to reduce or   50
prevent obesity

Table 7.1   Personalized medicine   58

Table 7.2   Incentives used to improve chronic care in European   63
             countries

Table 7.3   Recent policy initiatives to improve coordination and   72–73
             quality of chronic care

Table 7.4   Evidence of effectiveness: clinical decision support system 77–78
             (CDSS)

Figures

Fig. 1.1   Structure of the book   2

Fig. 2.1   Worldwide share of deaths by causes and countries within   11
             different World Bank income categories (2002)

Fig. 2.2   Burden of death and disease attributable to stroke in   14
             selected countries in the WHO European Region (2004)

Fig. 2.3   Burden of death and disease attributable to diabetes in   14
             selected countries in the WHO European Region (2004)

Fig. 2.4   Burden of death and disease attributable to COPD in   15
             selected countries in the WHO European Region (2004)

Fig. 2.5   Burden of disease attributable to unipolar depressive disorder 16
             in selected countries in the WHO European Region (2004)

Fig. 4.1   Prevention and stages of disease   27

Fig. 7.1   Financial relations between stakeholders in health care   61

Fig. 7.2   Types of care provision with varying degrees of   68
             coordination

Fig. 7.3   ELSID – study design   83

Boxes

Box 4.1   Disease management: key elements   34

Box 7.1   Structural barriers to coordination   69

List of abbreviations

AIDS	Acquired immunodeficiency syndrome
AOK	General regional health funds
BMI	Body mass index
CAD	Coronary artery disease
CCM	Chronic Care Model
CDSS	Clinical decision support system
CHF	Congestive heart failure
COPD	Chronic obstructive pulmonary disease
DALY	Disability-adjusted life year
DMP	Disease management programme
DNA	Deoxyribonucleic acid
DRG	Diagnosis-related group
ELSID	Evaluation of a Large-Scale Implementation of Disease Management Programs
EU	European Union
GDP	Gross domestic product
GINA	Global Initiative for Asthma
GP	General practitioner
HIV	Human immunodeficiency virus
HPV	Human papilloma virus
HRQoL	Health-related quality of life
HTA	Health technology assessment
ICT	Information and communication technology

NHS	National Health Service
OECD	Organisation for Economic Co-operation and Development
PAL	Physical activity level
PCT	Primary Care Trust
PUFA	Polyunsaturated fatty acids
QALYs	Quality-adjusted life years
QOF	Quality and Outcomes Framework
RCT	Randomized controlled trial
WHO	World Health Organization

About the authors

Reinhard Busse is Professor and Director of the Department of Health Care Management at the Berlin University of Technology, Germany, and Associate Head for Research Policy of the European Observatory on Health Systems and Policies.

Miriam Blümel, David Scheller-Kreinsen and **Annette Zentner** are research fellows at the Department of Health Care Management at the Berlin University of Technology, Germany.

Chapter 1
Introduction

Chronic diseases are the leading cause of mortality and morbidity in Europe, and research suggests that complex conditions such as diabetes and depression will impose an even larger burden in the future. Some years ago chronic diseases were considered to be a problem of the rich and elderly population. Today we know that within high-income countries, poor as well as young and middle-aged people are affected by chronic conditions. The economic implications of such diseases are also serious. Chronic diseases depress wages, earnings, workforce participation and labour productivity, as well as increasing early retirement, high job turnover and disability. Disease-related impairment of household consumption and educational performance has a negative effect on gross domestic product (GDP). As expenditure on chronic care rises across Europe, it takes up increasingly greater proportions of public and private budgets.

Chronic diseases have traditionally included the following: cardiovascular disease, diabetes and asthma or chronic obstructive pulmonary disease (COPD). As survival rates and durations have improved, this type of disease now also included many varieties of cancer, HIV/AIDS, mental disorders (such as depression, schizophrenia and dementia) and disabilities such as sight impairment and arthroses. Many chronic diseases and conditions are linked to an ageing society, but also to lifestyle choices such as smoking, sexual behaviour, diet and exercise, as well as to genetic predispositions.

What these diseases have in common is that they need a long-term and complex response, coordinated by different health professionals with access to the necessary drugs and equipment, and extending into social care. Most health care today, however, is still structured around acute episodes.

Given this background, the management of chronic disease is increasingly considered an important issue by policy-makers and researchers. Policy-makers across Europe are searching for interventions and strategies to tackle chronic disease. The World Health Organization (WHO) defines chronic disease management as the "ongoing management of conditions over a period of years or decades".

In 2008 the European Observatory on Health Systems and Policies published two important contributions. First, the book *Caring for people with chronic conditions: A health system perspective* edited by Ellen Nolte and Martin McKee greatly enhanced our understanding of the systematic dimensions of policy-making in the field of chronic disease. This is accompanied by the publication *Managing chronic conditions: Experience in eight countries*, edited by Ellen Nolte, Cécile Knai and Martin McKee, which provides in-depth case studies of policy-making with regard to chronic conditions in eight Organisation for Economic Co-operation and Development (OECD) countries.

This book aims to complement the two above-mentioned volumes by focusing more explicitly on the strategies and interventions that policy-makers have at their disposal to tackle chronic diseases.

The book consists of three parts (Fig. 1.1). The first sets the scene by outlining the burden of chronic disease on patients, groups and societies in Europe. Chapter 2 focuses on the epidemiologic burden of chronic disease and related risk factors in Europe and shows that chronic diseases are no longer confined to the old and rich. Chapter 3 outlines the economic implications of chronic diseases. We distinguish between results generated by microeconomic and macroeconomic analyses.

Fig. 1.1 *Structure of the book*

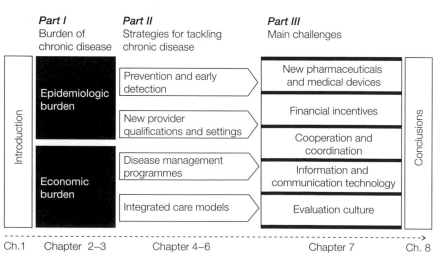

The second part of the book concentrates on strategies and interventions that policy-makers can use to tackle chronic diseases, in particular:

- prevention and early detection
- new provider qualifications and settings
- disease management programmes (DMPs)
- integrated care models.

Chapter 4 describes these strategies. Chapter 5 summarizes the evidence on effectiveness and Chapter 6 presents the evidence on cost–effectiveness. We find that most countries in Europe are applying various approaches of **disease prevention and early detection**. Prevention includes primary, secondary or tertiary approaches that differ in aims and target groups. Research indicates that broad approaches combining several interventions are most effective. From outside Europe, New Zealand's diabetes prevention programme is an example of a successful multilevel approach. Many prevention programmes tackle tobacco, alcohol consumption, obesity or hypertension. Cost–effectiveness for tobacco control is clear, but results of interventions to reduce and prevent obesity are inconclusive. Overall, analyses indicate that efficient strategies for prevention and early detection are available for many chronic conditions. Nevertheless, policy-makers have to be cautious: cost–effectiveness varies considerably according to regional context and different populations. This means that for each intervention they must examine carefully regional factors and specifically define their target groups. Overall, prevention and early detection programmes are promising, but far from well developed in most countries. Given the severe medical, social and economic consequences of chronic diseases, more effort and resources need to be invested in prevention.

Furthermore, the book shows that nearly all health care systems have recently seen the emergence of **new providers, settings and qualifications**. Once it became clear that traditional demarcation lines between physicians and nurses could harm quality of care, new professions – such as nurse practitioners, liaison nurses and community nurses – were set up. The tasks and responsibilities of existing professional groups have been shifted and expanded. For example, physicians now have a coordinating role by guiding patients through the health system. Since the late 1990s new ways of providing services have been set up. Collaborative models – such as group practices, medical polyclinics and nurse-led clinics – are more patient oriented. A key challenge is to support health workers in carrying out their new duties and responsibilities. There is a need for well-targeted training, particularly for those at the lower levels of the professional hierarchy. Evidence on these new qualifications and settings is limited, but pilot studies suggest that primary care nurses with more qualifications and responsibilities provide better care. New qualifications, structures and settings can help to improve the management of chronic diseases. Nevertheless, future research must build on these early results to see whether improvements justify investment, and also to inform future decisions.

Moreover, **DMPs** have been introduced by many European countries to improve chronic care and contain costs. The aim is to improve coordination by focusing on the whole care process, building on scientific evidence and patient involvement. Nevertheless, there are still insufficient rigorously designed large-scale population-based evaluations, but smaller studies suggest that these programmes may improve care. Several studies have shown the benefits of providers following evidence-based guidelines. Patients' behaviour has also changed, as indicated by greater patient satisfaction and adherence to treatment. Generally, the evidence suggests an improvement in the care process. The evidence on medical outcomes, however, is still inconclusive. Only a few studies have shown that DMPs affect mortality and other health-related outcomes. The evidence on cost–effectiveness is similarly inconclusive. Economic evaluation studies look only at costs and do not consider the relation of costs and benefits. Providers and insurers must make the data they collect available for research, and evaluation become an integral part of these programmes.

Finally, we find that **integrated care models** respond to the fact that chronic diseases can rarely be treated in isolation. Patients often have several chronic diseases or conditions at a time and need care from different providers. These models organize treatment (and prevention) so that services are better integrated across the whole range of care. Examples in Europe are the introduction of case management by the National Health Service (NHS) in the United Kingdom, and the pilot projects in Spain in which the whole care process is provided from only one source. All across Europe, various forms of provider networks and interventions have been set up to close the gap between primary and hospital services. Between 2004 and 2008, 1% of all payments for physicians and hospitals were earmarked for investing in integrated care projects. The effectiveness of these projects remains uncertain because so far the evidence is limited. Several components – such as self-management support, delivery system design and decision support – seem to be effective, but there is a lack of large-scale population-based studies. Some of the preliminary results give cause for optimism but, given the complexity of integrated care models, implementation will be challenging and future studies should focus on this. As far as cost–effectiveness is concerned, early results are inconclusive. Policy-makers must ensure that costs, savings and benefits are studied in more detail.

In the final section of the book (Chapter 7) we draw conclusions about important challenges to tackling chronic disease in Europe. It builds on the insights generated in Chapters 4, 5 and 6. It also outlines the conditions we identify for successful implementation of the main strategies and interventions.

In particular, our analysis suggests that **new pharmaceuticals and medical devices** can help to improve treatment for the chronically ill, but will bring new difficulties in terms of marketing authorization and reimbursement.

Moreover, we argue that properly applied **financial incentives** can be powerful tools to bring about effective and rapid change. However, policy-makers need to pay attention to operational aspects, such as the size of variable compensation or funding, as well as issues relating to goal-setting. In terms of chronic care, benefits tend to become apparent only after several years, which means that policy-makers must realize that often the quality of care will only be improved if providers are confident that they will be able to benefit from their investments. Hence, they need to look carefully at which strategy to follow with regard to **continuity of care**.

In addition, policy-makers should recognize that reforms intended to improve **coordination** must be well prepared and supported by strong political will. They should map out clearly the responsibilities of all the individuals and groups involved. The balance between local autonomy and central authority must be carefully defined. Policy-makers will also need to provide enough funding to enable reform, while at the same time setting up compensation schemes that will encourage professional groups to cooperate. Finally, health workers need adequate training and mutual learning and communication.

Furthermore, to release the full potential of **information and communication technology** (ICT), agreement must be reached on international technical standards. Solutions must be found for translating the vast amounts of data into meaningful information that health professionals can use.

Finally, **evaluation** should be an integral part of programmes to improve the management of chronic disease. The process should not block effective patient-oriented innovations, which is a dilemma for which new approaches need to be developed and agreed. Because policy-makers need better evidence in order to make informed decisions, existing data should immediately be made available for research.

Chapter 8 summarizes our findings and highlights some future research needs.

Part I
Burden of chronic disease

This part of the book outlines the burden of chronic disease on patients, groups and societies in Europe. Chapter 2 focuses on the epidemiology of chronic diseases and related risk factors in Europe. Chapter 3 examines the economic implications.

Chapter 2

Deaths and burden of chronic disease in Europe

This chapter looks at how chronic disease affect European countries in different ways. We examine mortality and the burden of disease across countries and regions, the prevalence of risk factors (such as smoking and being overweight) and the varying burdens of selected chronic conditions. Finally, we estimate the future mortality and burden of chronic disease.

2.1 Current status

The burden of chronic diseases

WHO defines chronic diseases as "diseases of long duration and generally slow progression". Often, the terms "noncommunicable disease" and "chronic disease" are treated as interchangeable, but given recent advances in treating communicable diseases this use is no longer precise enough. For example, HIV/ AIDS treated with modern medicines has become a disease of long duration and generally slow progression. We acknowledge this issue, but nevertheless refer to sources that use noncommunicable disease as a proxy for chronic disease if no alternative high-quality data are available. Following the WHO classification, cancer is treated as a chronic disease in this book, even though it is acknowledged that the strategies used in chronic disease management are not always applicable to patients with this disease.

Chronic disease is responsible for most of the disease and deaths in Europe. One measure of the overall burden of disease, developed by WHO, is the disability-adjusted life year (DALY). It is designed to quantify the impact on a population of premature death and disability by combining them into a single measure. The DALY relies on the assumption that the most appropriate measure of the effects of chronic illness is time either spent disabled by disease or lost due to premature death. One DALY equals one year of healthy life lost (WHO 2005).

Table 2.1 shows the number of both DALYs and deaths, as well as their percentage as a share of all causes in 2005 (Singh 2008; WHO 2005). In the same year, cardiovascular diseases were the cause of 5.07 million or 52% of all deaths – with a disease burden of 34.42 million DALYs.

Table 2.1 *Disease burden and deaths from noncommunicable diseases in the WHO European Region by cause (2005)*

Groups of causes	Disease burden		Deaths	
	DALYs (millions)	Proportion from all causes (%)	Number (millions)	Proportion from all causes (%)
Selected noncommunicable diseases				
Cardiovascular diseases	34.42	23	5.07	52
Neuropsychiatric conditions	29.37	20	0.26	3
Cancer (malignant neoplasms)	17.03	11	1.86	19
Digestive diseases	7.12	5	0.39	4
Respiratory diseases	6.84	5	0.42	4
Sense organ diseases	6.34	4	0	0
Musculoskeletal diseases	5.75	4	0.03	0
Diabetes mellitus	2.32	2	0.15	2
Oral conditions	1.02	1	0	2
All noncommunicable diseases	*115.34*	*77*	*8.21*	*86*
All causes	*150.32*	*100*	*9.56*	*100*

Source: Adapted from Singh 2008.

The incidence of chronic diseases is high in high-income countries. The WHO's project **The Global Burden of Disease** estimates incidence, prevalence, severity and duration, and mortality for more than 130 major causes. It includes data since 2000 for WHO member countries and for subregions throughout the world (WHO 2008a; WHO 2008b; WHO 2009). Fig. 2.1 shows the high share of chronic or noncommunicable diseases compared with communicable, maternal, perinatal and nutritional conditions, as well as injuries in low-income, lower-middle income, upper-middle income and high-income countries (Suhrcke et al. 2006).[1]

---

[1] The four groups are according to the income categories used by the World Bank.

Fig. 2.1 *Worldwide share of deaths by causes and countries within different World Bank income categories (2002)*

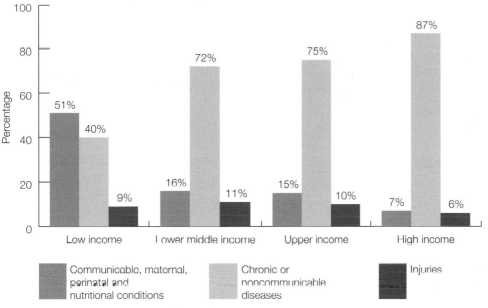

Sources: Suhrcke et al. 2006; Mathers et al. 2003.

The WHO project estimates that in 2002 chronic or noncommunicable conditions accounted for 87% of deaths in high-income countries (Fig. 2.1). Only 7% of deaths were attributed to communicable conditions and nutritional deficiencies and 6% to injuries (WHO 2005). The proportion of deaths worldwide caused by noncommunicable disease is projected to rise from 59% in 2002 to 69% in 2030 (Mathers and Loncar 2005).

Most studies focus on chronic conditions and on risk factors between countries, while only a few have looked at the distribution within countries. However, increasing data from high income countries almost unanimously show that the poor within these countries carry a higher chronic disease burden than the rich (Suhrcke et al. 2006).

The link between disease and age is also crucial from an economic and public policy standpoint. The proportion of those in European countries aged 65 years and older is projected to grow from 15% in 2000 to 23.5% by 2030. The proportion of those aged 80 years and over is expected to more than double from 3% in 2000 to 6.4% in 2030 (Pomerleau, Knai and Nolte 2008; Kinsella and Phillips 2005). This trend is clearly one of the reasons for the growing burden of chronic conditions and diseases.

Older people are not the only ones affected by chronic diseases. Rising numbers of young and middle-aged people have some form of chronic health problem

(Pomerleau, Knai and Nolte 2008). The above-mentioned WHO project estimated that 72% of all deaths before the age of 60 years in 2002 were due to chronic or noncommunicable conditions in high-income countries, whereas communicable diseases accounted for only 8% and injuries for 21%. In the same year, 68% of DALYs lost to chronic diseases in high-income countries occurred among those of working age. These findings suggest that chronic disease can no longer be considered just a problem of the elderly (Suhrcke et al. 2006; Mathers et al. 2003).

The burden of chronic disease risk factors

The shape of the future burden of chronic disease can be projected by data on risk factors (Suhrcke et al. 2006). Globally, the main risk factors for chronic disease are hypertension, tobacco use, high cholesterol, low fruit and vegetable intake, overweight and obesity, sedentary lifestyle and alcohol abuse. Except for low fruit and vegetable intake, all of them are relatively more important risk factors in high-income countries than in low- and middle-income countries; however, the majority of the deaths and the higher burden of disease are found in the latter. Table 2.2 presents deaths and DALYs attributable to risk factors; it shows that high blood pressure is responsible for 7.62 million deaths globally (13.5% of all deaths), of which 6.22 million occur in low- and middle-income countries and 1.39 million in high-income countries.

Table 2.2 *Deaths and burden of disease attributable to common risk factors, in absolute numbers and percentages of all deaths/DALYs, by contribution to worldwide deaths (2001)*

Chronic disease risk factors	Low- and middle-income		High-income		Worldwide	
	Deaths	DALYs	Deaths	DALYs	Deaths	DALYs
	(millions)		(millions)		(millions)	
High blood pressure	6.22 (12.9%)	78.06 (5.6%)	1.39 (17.6%)	13.89 (9.3%)	7.62 (13.5%)	91.95 (6.0%)
Smoking	3.34 (6.9%)	54.02 (3.9%)	1.46 (18.5%)	18.90 (12.7%)	4.80 (8.5%)	72.92 (4.7%)
High cholesterol	3.04 (6.3%)	42.82 (3.1%)	0.84 (10.7%)	9.43 (6.3%)	3.88 (6.9%)	52.25 (3.4%)
Low fruit and vegetable intake	2.31 (4.8%)	32.84 (2.4%)	0.33 (4.2%)	3.98 (2.7%)	2.64 (4.7%)	36.82 (2.4%)
Overweight and obesity	1.75 (3.6%)	31.52 (2.3%)	0.61 (7.8%)	10.73 (7.2%)	2.36 (4.2%)	42.25 (2.8%)
Physical inactivity	1.56 (3.2%)	22.68 (1.6%)	0.38 (4.8%)	4.73 (3.2%)	1.94 (3.4%)	27.41 (1.8%)

Source: Adapted from Lopez et al. 2006.

According to the WHO report *The world health report 2002 – Reducing risks, promoting healthy life* (and confirmed by data in Table 2.2), tobacco use still remains the leading avoidable cause of death in industrialized nations (WHO 2002). In Europe since the late 1970s the proportion of smokers has dropped from 45% to 30%. However, in eastern European countries, and particularly in the Baltic states, smoking has continued to increase, particularly among young people and women (Novotny 2008).

Alcohol abuse causes chronic illnesses, such as alcohol dependence, vascular disease (such as hypertension), cirrhosis and various cancers. Of the global loss of DALYs, 4.7% can be explained by alcohol-related diseases. At 10.7%, the share for eastern Europe is significantly higher (Jamison 2006; Novotny 2008).

Overweight is defined as a body mass index (BMI or kg/m^3) of 25 or more. People with a BMI of 30 or more are classified as obese. According to this definition, almost a third of all people living in Europe are overweight. Older age groups show higher prevalence (up to 57% of men in western Europe aged 70–79 years) (James et al. 2004; Novotny 2008). However, an increasing number of European children are affected: one study by the London Obesity Task Force found that 18% of children in Europe were overweight (Novotny 2008).

Variation of burden: selected chronic conditions in Europe

The contribution of chronic diseases to the overall mortality and burden of disease varies within Europe, as the leading chronic conditions illustrate. However, with some diseases we do not know how much of this variation is caused by disease, and how much by differences in coding by health professionals in the various countries (Pomerleau, Knai and Nolte 2008).

Cerebrovascular disease or **stroke** accounted for approximately 15% of all deaths (11% in men and 19% in women) and approximately 7% of total disease burden (6% and 8% respectively) in 2002 in Europe (WHO Regional Office for Europe 2004). However, the mortality and disease burden attributed to stroke in Europe varies considerably. The Russian Federation, Kyrgyzstan and Kazakhstan have up to 10 times higher levels than Switzerland, Israel and France (Fig 2.2).

Mortality and disease burden from **diabetes mellitus** also vary considerably (Fig. 2.3). Age-standardized death rates in 2004 ranged from below 4.0 per 100 000 in Ukraine, Belarus and Greece to 23.0 per 100 000 in Portugal, 31.8 per 100 000 in Israel and even 68.6 per 100 000 in Armenia. These figures however, are likely to be an underestimate because diabetes is not always recorded as the underlying cause of death, particularly for older people (Pomerleau, Knai and Nolte 2008). In addition, for some countries with apparently low death rates the burden of disease has been estimated to be above average.

Fig. 2.2 *Burden of death and disease attributable to stroke in selected countries in the WHO European region (2004)*

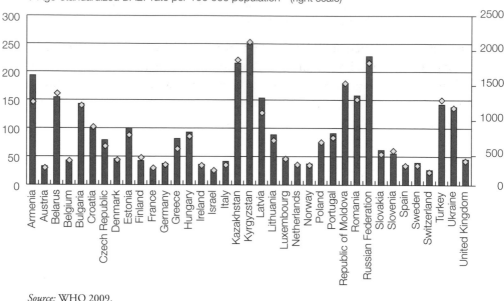

■ Age-standardized death rate per 100 000 population - (left scale)
◇ Age-standardized DALY rate per 100 000 population - (right scale)

Source: WHO 2009.

Fig. 2.3 *Burden of death and disease attributable to diabetes in selected countries in the WHO European Region (2004)*

■ Age-standardized death rate per 100 000 population - (left scale)
◇ Age-standardized DALY rate per 100 000 population - (right scale)

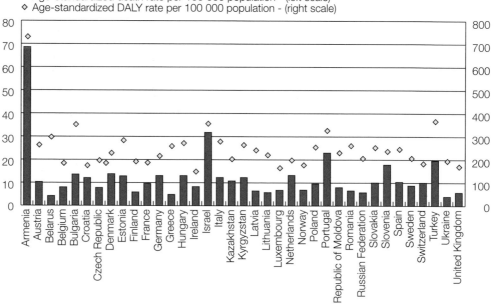

Source: WHO 2009.

Chronic obstructive pulmonery disease (COPD) is also one of the leading causes of premature death in Europe and its contribution varies considerably in different countries. In 2004, COPD was associated with an estimated 6.5 deaths and 91 DALYs per 100 000 population in Latvia, while in Kyrgyzstan it was associated with 96.0 deaths and 1363 DALYs per 100 000 (Fig. 2.4).

The prevalence of mental disorders is high in Europe (Kessler 2007). **Dementia** among those aged 65 years and over in 2000 was estimated to vary between 6% in eastern Europe and 8% in northern Europe (Wimo et al. 2003). More recent estimates have placed the prevalence of dementia among those aged 60 years and over at 3.8% in eastern Europe and 5.4% in western Europe (Ferri et al. 2005).

Fig. 2.4 *Burden of death and disease attributable to COPD in selected countries in the WHO European Region (2004)*

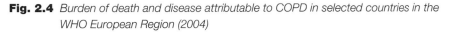

■ Age-standardized death rate per 100 000 population - (left scale)
◇ Age-standardized DALY rate per 100 000 population - (right scale)

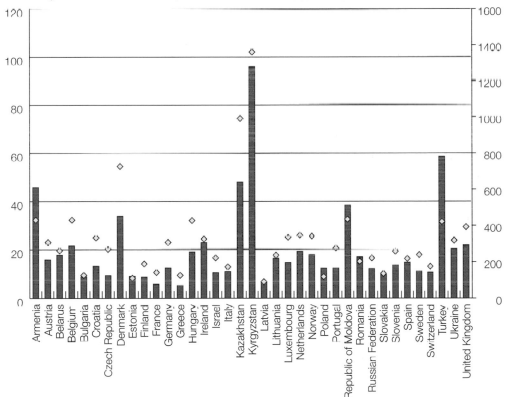

Source: WHO 2009.

WHO has estimated that one person in five will develop **depression** and that each year 33.4 million Europeans have major depression (WHO 2003). In 2004, age-adjusted DALY rates ranged from 620 to 1340 DALYs per 100 000 (Fig. 2.5). Rates were lowest in Spain, Greece and Portugal, with DALYs below 700 per 100 000. The highest estimates were for Finland, Israel, Slovenia, Belgium and France, with rates of more than 1200 DALYs per 100 000 (WHO 2009). Suicide from depressive disorders is the third leading cause of death among young people in Europe (Pomerleau, Knai and Nolte 2008).

Fig. 2.5 *Burden of disease attributable to unipolar depressive disorder in selected countries in the WHO European Region (2004)*

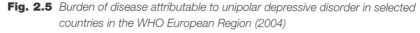

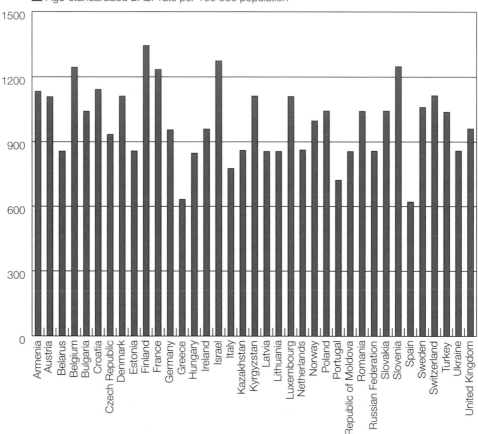

Source: WHO 2009.

2.2 Predictions

Baseline predictions

Projections of future mortality and burden of disease show that chronic diseases will continue to be the biggest contributor to mortality and disability in high–income countries, and chronic disease will increase. The share of DALYs associated with chronic or noncommunicable conditions in high-income countries is projected to rise from 86% in 2005 to 89% in 2030 (Suhrcke et al. 2006; Mathers and Loncar 2005).

Predictions for selected chronic conditions in Europe

Predictions for specific chronic conditions vary. For example, WHO has projected fewer deaths (−1%) and DALYs (−17%) from stroke for both sexes and across all ages in Europe between 2008 and 2030 (WHO 2008b). In contrast, Carandang, Seshadri and Beiser (2006), while agreeing that both incidence and mortality are declining, argue for a higher prevalence, and therefore burden of disease, due to improvements in stroke treatment and an ageing population prone to strokes.

Deaths directly attributable to diabetes are predicted to rise from about 166 000 in 2009 to over 209 000 in 2030 (WHO 2008b). The growth of diabetes type 2 is partly a result of rising obesity levels, especially among children (Pomerleau, Knai and Nolte 2008).

Deaths in Europe from COPD are expected to rise by about 20%, from 248 000 in 2008 to more than 300 000 in 2030 (WHO 2008b). Despite these predictions, the burden of COPD is projected to fall from about 2.91 million to 2.57 million DALYs (WHO 2008b). However, the death rate and DALYs attributable to COPD are expected to decrease in all groups other than women aged 70 years and older (Pomerleau, Knai and Nolte 2008).

Unipolar depressive disorders are projected to fall slightly between 2005 and 2030. WHO has projected a decrease in age-standardized death rates from 0.15 to 0.13 per 100 000. However, the burden of disease attributatble to this problem is projected to increase among men from 777 to 785 per 100 000 (1%) and among women by 1.8% (from 1312 to 1337 per 100 000) (Pomerleau, Knai and Nolte 2008).

The condition expected to increase most dramatically is dementia. The number of those in Europe aged 60 years and over with dementia is estimated to rise from 7.7 million in 2001 to 10.8 million in 2020. Without effective prevention and treatment, this is expected to double to 15.9 million in 2040. The increase varies between 31% and 51% in different regions (Ferri et al. 2005).

Chapter 3
Economic consequences of chronic disease

There is considerable evidence on the epidemiology of chronic disease, but little on its economic implications. This chapter reviews recent microeconomic and macroeconomic evidence. The economic implications of specific strategies should not be the main or only guide when making health care decisions, but one purpose of any intervention must be to improve health cost-effectively. Clearly, policy-makers often target economic variables such as cost savings, greater labour productivity or economic growth, but these should not be the main criteria for evaluating specific strategies in chronic disease management. In order to understand the implications of chronic conditions and diseases, the economic implications should be examined.

3.1 The microeconomic perspective

Microeconomics examines the consequences of chronic disease on individuals and households. The key routes through which ill health in general, and chronic diseases in particular, may impact on the economy, are through its effects on consumption and savings (capital formation), labour productivity and supply as well as education (Suhrcke et al. 2005). The evidence from European countries is growing but still limited (Suhrcke et al. 2008). So far it has identified various effects of chronic conditions, explored here (Suhrcke et al. 2006).

Treating chronic diseases may be particularly costly in countries where a high share of total health spending is paid "out of pocket". Spending on addictive products such as tobacco and alcohol may cause poor health, and the household's ability to keep consumption levels constant in the face of "health shocks" can be very costly.

With regard to **labour supply and labour productivity**, chronic conditions and diseases mean fewer people in the workforce, with early retirement, barriers to employment, and stigma. There is reasonable evidence on the negative impact of chronic disease and risk factors on the labour market, showing that chronic disease affects labour supply in terms of workforce participation, hours worked, job turnover and early retirement (Table 3.1) as well as wages, earnings and position reached (Table 3.2).

Table 3.1 *Impact of chronic diseases and conditions and risk factors on labour supply, selected examples*

Country and study	Year data collected	Chronic diseases and conditions and impact of these on employment indicators/labour supply
Canada Kraut et al. 2001	1983–1990	Diabetes Affected people 2.1-fold less likely to work
Europe Jimenez-Martin et al. 1999	1994–1995	Chronic disease Chronic disease increases the retirement probability Husband's health affects the couple's retirement decisions much more strongly than the wife's health does
Finland Sarlio-Lahteenko-rva and Lahelma 1999	1994	Obesity Women face a 2.5-fold higher likelihood of unemployment Women face a 1.4-fold higher likelihood of unemployment
Ireland Gannon and Nolan 2004	2000	Chronic disease Men 61% less likely to work; women 52% less likely to work
	2002	Chronic disease Men 66% less likely to work; women 42% less likely to work
Russian Federation Suhrcke, Rocco and McKee 2007b	2002	Chronic disease Retirement age decreases by 2.5 years Men have a 13.6% greater chance of retirement Women have a 14.0% greater chance of retirement
Sweden Lindholm et al. 2001	1979–1997	Chronic disease Unemployment 1.9-fold higher 2.5-fold increase in people receiving welfare benefits 1.8-fold increase in people with financial difficulties 3.5-fold increase in economic inactivity
United States Serxner et al. 2001	1990–1998	Mental health Absenteeism is 47% higher
		Tobacco use Absenteeism is 19% higher
		Obesity Absenteeism is 23% higher
United States Simon et al. 2000	n/a	Depression 15.3% higher employment rate for depression remission versus control group

Table 3.1 *cont.*

United States Dwyer and Mitch- ell 1999	1992	Cardiovascular disease Expected retirement age decreases by 0.7 years
		High blood pressure Expected retirement age decreases by 1.0 year
		Diabetes Expected retirement age decreases by 0.12 years
		Cancer Expected retirement age decreases by 0.13 years
United States Pelkowski and Berger 2004	1992–1993	Chronic disease Men work 6.1% fewer hours Women work 3.9% fewer hours
United States McGarry 2002	1992–1994	Self-reported adult health Men 3.5% less likely to work at age 62
United States Coile 2003	1992–2000	Chronic disease Men have a 42% greater probability of retirement and lose 1030 hours of lifetime work Women have a 31% probability of retirement and lose 654 hours of lifetime work
United States Cawley 2004	1997–2004	Obesity For white people, a 10% weight increase corresponds to a 12% decrease in probability of full-time employment, 5.4% fewer hours worked, 5% fewer months, 16% increase in months receiving welfare benefits, and 10% lower earnings. For African American people, a 10% weight gain corresponds to a 10.9% increase in months spent receiving welfare benefits

Source: Suhrcke et al. 2006
Note: n/a: Not available.

Table 3.2 *Impact of chronic diseases and conditions and risk factors on wages, earnings or incomes, selected examples*

Country and study	Year data collected	Chronic diseases and conditions and impact of these on employment Indicators/labour supply
Australia Lee 1999	1980–1989	Tobacco use Wages are 6.6% lower for smokers and 5.5% lower for former smokers
Canada Kraut et al. 2001	1983–1990	Diabetes Wages decrease by 28%
Canada Auld 1998	1991	Tobacco use Daily smokers earn 30% less than non-smokers
Finland Sarlio- Lahteenkorva and Lahelma 1999	1994	Obesity Likelihood of low household income increases by 1.5 times Likelihood of low individual income increases by 1.6 times
Indonesia Kosen 1998 (unpublished report)	1995	Tobacco use Lost annual income is US$115 for individuals who use tobacco Lost annual income is also US$115 for family members of tobacco users

Table 3.2 *cont.*

Netherlands Van Ours 2004	2001	Tobacco use Wages 10% lower
Russian Federation Suhrcke, Rocco and McKee 2007b	2002	Chronic disease 5.6% lower median per-person income
United Kingdom Sargent and Blanchflower 1994	1974–1981	Obesity Wages reduced by 6.4% for 23-year-old women
United States Tucker and Friedman 1998	n/a	Obesity Likelihood of absenteeism increases 1.7-fold for men Likelihood of absenteeism increases 1.6-fold for women
United States Pronk et al. 2004	n/a	Obesity Obese employees are less likely to get along with co-workers and more likely to incur lost work days
		Physical activity Physical activity was positively associated with the quality of work performed and overall job performance
		Cardiac fitness Cardio-respiratory fitness is positively associated with the quantity of work performed, and with extra effort exerted at work
United States Fielding 1996	n/a	Physical inactivity Productivity declined 50% in the last two hours of work each day
United States Sloan et al. 2004	n/a	Tobacco use Lifetime wages reduced by US$40 000
United States Gortmaker et al. 1993	1981–1988	Obesity Income for men is 9% lower (equivalent to a reduction of US$2876) Income for women is 22% lower (US$6710)
United States Cawley 2004	1981–2000	Obesity For white females, a difference in weight of two standard deviations (roughly 65 pounds) is associated with a difference in wages of 9% (in absolute value, this is equivalent to the wage effect of roughly one and a half years of education or three years of work experience)
United States Levine et al. 1997	1984–1992	Tobacco use Wages decrease by 4–8%
United States Zagorsky 2004	1985–2000	Obesity An increase in BMI of one point reduces net worth by US$1000
United States Bhattacharya and Bundorf 2004	1989–1998	Obesity Wages reduced by US$0.71 per hour
United States Haskins and Ransford 1999	1988 and 1998	Obesity Higher weight tends to lower the chances for women to enter higher professional or managerial positions

Table 3.2 *cont.*

United States Ng et al. 2001	1989	Diabetes 3% reduction in wages (US$3700–8700 per year)
United States Averett and Korenman 1999	1990	Obesity White women's wages are reduced by 17%
United States Pelkowski and Berger 2004	1992–1993	Chronic disease Men earn 5.6% less; women earn 8.9% less
United States Mitra 2001	1993	Obesity Women earn US$1.26 less per hour One pound increase in weight is associated with 2% decrease in wages for women in professional/managerial positions
United States Berndt et al. 2000	1995	Depression 12–18% lower wages over lifetime

Source: Suhrcke et al.2006.
Note: n/a: Not available.

Suhrcke et al. have recently added to this body of evidence on the effects on the labour market by adding empirical data on Albania, Bosnia and Herzegovina, Bulgaria, Estonia, Kosovo[2], Tajikistan and Ukraine (data here not shown, please refer to Suhrcke, Rocco and McKee 2007a pp. 109–119).

Education and human capital formation are accepted as a powerful determinant of future earnings and future health. A full assessment of the costs of chronic disease should include the impact on education; current evidence shows that it affects educational performance. The death of a parent can reduce school enrolment (Gertler, Levine and Ames 2004). Several studies have reported an association between maternal smoking and impaired cognitive and behavioural development, which in turn affects the academic performance of children (Ernst, Moolchan and Robinson 2001). Alcohol abuse is related to poor performance. This applies to young people in developed countries, where excessive drinking among younger age groups is relatively widespread (Suhrcke et al. 2006). Overweight or obese children are more likely to suffer from low self-esteem as a result of stigmatization and this leads to absence from school (Latner and Stunkard 2003; Hayden-Wade et al. 2005).

The effects of chronic conditions and diseases on labour market outcomes and education are especially pronounced in low- and middle-income countries. In Europe, health insurance mitigates some of these effects. Nevertheless, the consequences remain negative in terms of the impact on labour supply, productivity, education and the accumulation of human capital.

---

[2] In accordance with Security Council resolution 1244 (1999).

Overall, the evidence shows that chronic conditions and diseases have a negative effect on the labour market and on the formation of human capital. However, the causal linkages are far from clear and these gaps need to be filled by further research.

3.2 The macroeconomic perspective

The macroeconomic perspective looks at the overall effect in terms of GDP or the GDP growth rate.

Health – as measured by life expectancy or adult mortality – is a robust predictor of economic growth. As shown in Chapter 2, chronic disease constitutes a major part of the global health burden. Mortality, DALYs and reduced life expectancy from chronic disease can be expected to depress economic growth. However, research on this has been limited, partly as a result of data and methodological challenges (Suhrcke et al. 2006).

There is evidence that health is a significant determinant of economic growth for high-income countries. A study by Barro (1996) estimated that a 5-year advantage in life expectancy explains a 0.3–0.5% higher annual GDP growth rate in subsequent years. Although this study does not focus on chronic disease, these results suggest a significant relationship between health and growth.

More recently, Suhrcke and Urban (2006) found that cost-of-illness studies showed that the cost of chronic diseases and their risk factors had a sizeable impact on a country's GDP, ranging from 0.02% to 6.77%. They looked at the worldwide impact of cardiovascular mortality on economic growth among the working-age population. In high-income countries, they found that a 1% increase in the mortality rate decreased the growth rate of per capita income in the following five years by approximately 0.1%. This may appear a small figure in terms of growth, but it becomes quite substantial when calculated over the long term (Suhrcke, Fahey and McKee 2008).

PART II
Strategies for tackling chronic disease

Part II examines the strategies and interventions available to tackle chronic disease. Chapter 4 describes them. Chapter 5 presents evidence on the effectiveness of each of the four strategies, and Chapter 6 summarizes the evidence on cost–effectiveness.

Chapter 4

Strategies against chronic disease: what is being done?

In this chapter we describe strategies for tackling chronic disease, looking at countries that have innovated. These include a range of European countries, as well as Canada, Australia, New Zealand and the United States. They provide important and useful lessons.

4.1 Prevention and early detection

Most countries are experimenting with disease prevention and early detection. Prevention includes primary, secondary or tertiary approaches that differ in aims and target groups (Fig. 4.1).

Fig. 4.1 Prevention and stages of disease

Course of disease	A	B	C	D
	Primary	Secondary prevention		Tertiary
A–B	Period of increased risk			
B	First observable pathophysiological changes			
C	First changes perceivable by patient			
D	Course can no longer be influenced			

Primary prevention is directed at the prevention of illnesses by removing the causes. The target group for primary prevention is those that are healthy with respect to the target disease.

Secondary prevention aims at identifying the disease at an early stage so that it can be treated. This makes an early cure possible (or at least the prevention of further deterioration). The target group for secondary prevention consists of people who are already ill without being aware of it, or those who have an increased risk or a genetic disposition.

Tertiary prevention is directed toward people who are already known to suffer from an illness. This is therefore a form of care. Tertiary prevention includes activities intended to cure, to ameliorate or to compensate. For example, the avoidance of complications of the prevention of progress of disease would be classed as tertiary prevention.

Source: Van der Maas and Mackenbach 1999.

The approaches vary according to the health care system and the dominant political opinions involved. Different countries may place different emphasis on the responsibility of the community and the individual, depending on cultural views regarding the role of the state and individual autonomy (Busse and Schlette 2007).

Scandinavian policies, for example, attach considerable importance to environmental factors and social conditions. Other countries, such as France, Germany and the United States focus more on the individual's attitude to risk factors such as tobacco, alcohol and nutrition (Busse, Zentner and Schlette 2006).

Some countries, such as the United Kingdom, Canada and New Zealand, emphasize integrated approaches, with clinical care systems as part of a broader approach that involves public health and health promotion efforts linked to disease management and support for self-care (Novotny 2008). The following subsection gives an overview of the different prevention strategies.

Tobacco and alcohol interventions

Increasingly more European countries have been tackling tobacco consumption and its negative health consequences (Busse and Schlette 2007). Common elements are:

- **pricing policies**: taxes, minimum duties and minimum prices;
- **information and communication**: limits on advertising and promotion, product displays and marketing, and requirements for compulsory labelling;
- **packaging**: minimum size of packs of cigarettes;
- **distribution**: restriction on sales to minors, introduction of cigarette vending machines with youth protection technology;
- **consumption**: smoking bans in public places, bars and restaurants and in the workplace; and
- **smoking cessation**: behavioural assistance.

Similar policies have been developed for alcohol abuse. Raising prices with higher taxes does reduce consumption. Bans on advertising are thought to reduce social acceptance of excess drinking. Sales of alcohol may be restricted to licensed retail outlets or during limited hours, and minimum age restrictions applied. Strict driving laws discourage excessive drinking and prevent traffic accidents (Novotny 2008).

Obesity interventions

There are various approaches to preventing obesity. These include public information and disclosure, targeting children and adolescents, taxing unhealthy food, planning the urban environment, and food prohibitions (Novotny 2008).

The dominant approach in obesity control is primary prevention. The European Commission has developed an action plan for European dietary guidelines based on existing evidence on health promotion programmes. The plan describes population goals in terms of nutrients and lifestyle for the prevention of chronic diseases in Europe (European Commission 2000). Table 4.1 sets out the components, goals and levels of evidence criteria.

Table 4.1 *Population goals for nutrients and features of lifestyle consistent with the prevention of major public health problems in Europe*

Component	Population goals	Levels of evidence
Physical activity levels (PAL)	1.75	++
BMI (kg/m³)	21–22	++
Dietary fat as % of total energy	<30	++
Fatty acids as % of total energy		
Saturated	<10	++++
Trans	<2	++
Polyunsaturated (PUFA)		
n-6	4–8	+++
n-3	2g linoleic + 200 mg very long chain	++
Carbohydrates as % of total energy	>55	+++
Sugary food consumption occasions per day	≤4	++
Fruit and vegetables (g/d)	>400	++
Folate from food (µg/d)	>400	+++
Dietary fibre (g/d)	>25 (or 3g/MJ)	++
Sodium (expressed as sodium chloride) (g/d)	<6	+++
Iodine (µg/d)	150 (infants 50; in pregnancy 200)	+++
Exclusive breastfeeding	About 6 months	+++

Source: European Commission 2000.
Notes: Levels of evidence: (++++) multiple double blind placebo controlled trials; (+++) single study of double blind analyses (breastfeeding – series of non-double blind analyses); (++) ecological analyses compatible with non-double blind intervention and physiological studies; (+) integration of multiple levels of evidence by expert groups.

Although there are effective interventions to reduce obesity, in many countries the response to the challenge is inadequate. For example, few European nations have average diets containing less than 30% of dietary energy from fat (Novotny 2008).

Hypertension interventions

It is widely agreed that effective approaches to hypertension should be combined with other strategies aimed at reducing risk factors for ischaemic heart disease (Novotny 2008). Such programmes in Europe and elsewhere include weight loss, healthy diet (high in potassium and low in sodium, low fat, adequate fruit and vegetable consumption), physical activity and moderate alcohol consumption (Chobanian et al. 2003).

Examples of specific intervention programmes

The international trend is towards holistic approaches to prevention. For example, the national diabetes prevention programme in New Zealand (Busse, Zentner and Schlettte 2006) combines primary, secondary and tertiary approaches and thus reaches the whole target population. The programme has the following 10 fields of action with specific goals and measures for each (CHSRP et al. 2006), in which representatives of various sectors – such as local government, the food industry, cultural groups, schools, sports clubs, and public and private health institutions – are working together:

1. supporting community leadership and action;

2. promoting behaviour change through social marketing;

3. changing urban design to support healthy and active lifestyles;

4. supporting a healthy environment through cooperation with the food industry;

5. strengthening health promotion;

6. improving well-child services;

7. working with schools to ensure children are "fit, healthy and ready to learn";

8. supporting primary care prevention and early intervention;

9. enabling vulnerable families to make healthy choices;

10. improving service integration and care for those with advanced disease(s).

Similarly, New Zealand's strategy against cancer highlights the fact that every public health strategy should try to integrate all aspects of the population's health, to implement programmes across different sectors, and to bring together all those involved. The cancer control strategy has six goals (CHSRP 2005):

1. preventing lifestyle-related, infectious and work-related health risks;

2. ensuring effective screening programmes;

3. ensuring effective diagnosis and treatment;

4. improving quality of life for cancer patients and their families through social support, rehabilitation and palliative care;

5. improving the delivery of services for all types of cancer care; and

6. improving the effectiveness of cancer control through research and surveillance.

For all sectors, the action plan for 2005–2010 determined secondary goals, defined target outcomes, specified steps for actions and established "milestones".

The British Government formulated a national cancer plan in 2000, specifying targets and standards for prevention, medical care and palliative medicine. Since 2006 this has included a national screening programme for bowel cancer, which pilot studies suggest has been successful (Oliver 2005).

European measures to prevent specific chronic diseases also include vaccination. For example, the approval of the human papilloma virus (HPV) vaccine to prevent cervical cancer in Europe is now part of immunization programmes in Austria, Germany, France and Italy (limited by age and sex), Belgium, Luxembourg, Norway, Sweden, Switzerland and the United Kingdom (Arun 2007).

4.2 New provider qualifications and settings

Chronic diseases increase the complexity of health problems and the provision of care, requiring changes in professional activities, qualifications and care settings. This section examines new approaches in terms of provider qualifications and settings.

New provider qualifications

Physicians play a key role in guiding patients through the health system and therefore need to be trained to coordinate activities. In the Spanish region of Castile and León, medical and social services for chronic care have been integrated. Ensuring that physicians were appropriately qualified was found to be a major precondition (Casado 2003). Australia, the United Kingdom and the Scandinavian countries have used "collaborative methodology" by training physicians to play a guiding role (Haas 2005). This methodology was developed in the 1990s by the United States Institute for Healthcare Improvement and involves a learning system aimed at improving care in specific areas, such as asthma, diabetes, heart disease and cancer (Busse, Zentner and Schlette 2006).

Providers have also been experimenting with new types of care. Many countries are becoming convinced that the traditional demarcation lines between health professions – for example, between physicians and nurses – are harmful, and they are beginning to redistribute responsibilities. A new profession of **nurse practitioner** has been established in the United Kingdom, the Netherlands, the United States, Canada, Australia and New Zealand (Busse and Schlette 2007; CHSRP 2006; Van Dijk 2003; McIntosh 2006). These university-trained professionals carry out traditional nursing duties, but also assume responsibility for tasks that would traditionally be viewed as part of a doctor's remit, such as limited prescribing of pharmaceuticals and administering less complex treatments.

Germany has recently created **community nurses**, similar to nurse practitioners in other countries. They make house visits and are responsible for basic primary care, supported by eHealth equipment. This gives chronically ill people in rural regions better access to basic medical care. It also relieves family doctors for other work (Busse and Schlette 2007; Blum 2006).

Another new professional group comprises **liaison nurses**, introduced in several European countries. They carry out follow-ups after discharge, pulmonary rehabilitation for people with COPD, supervision of medication and compliance, patient education and service navigation. **Case managers** coordinate services for people with long-term conditions or with complex social and medical needs. Their functions include assessing people's needs, developing care plans, helping people access appropriate care, monitoring the quality of this care, and maintaining contact with the person and her/his family (Dubois, Singh and Jiwani 2008). In England, for example, case management is part of the strategy within all Primary Care Trusts (PCTs). These trusts provide primary medical care and community nursing services, and are taking over responsibility for purchasing secondary care. Other groups, such as pharmacists and social workers, have also been able to perform new roles. For instance, a contract introduced in England in 2004 enabled pharmacists to expand their role by providing repeat prescriptions, reviewing medication and compliance, and providing smoking cessation services (Dubois, Singh and Jiwani 2008). Hence, task sharing among health professionals aiming at efficient, effective clinical care has been integrated as a central idea in most policy approaches.

Last, but not least, the central role of **family caregivers** in monitoring, treating and managing chronic diseases and conditions is increasingly acknowledged (Wilkins, Bruce and Sirey 2009). Their role is expanding as the number of people with chronic conditions and disabilities accelerates, and changes in health care delivery – for example early discharge in the hospital sector – emphasize care in private settings (Edwards et al. 2002). The importance of family caregivers has been extensively demonstrated for various illnesses, such as dementia (Gallagher-Thompson and Coon 2007), heart failure (Bakas et al. 2006), stroke (Grant et al. 2004), depression (McCusker et al. 2007) and various other diseases (Wilkins, Bruce and Sirey 2009). As a consequence, family caregivers have become a significant component of the health care "workforce" (Schumacher, Beck and Marren 2006). Family caregivers can be active in various institutional environments such as hospices (Haley et al. 2003), hospitals (Messecar, Powers and Nagel 2008) or private settings. Conceptually, the increasing acknowledgement of the importance of family caregivers is reflected by home health care models, which explicitly recognize them as powerful allies (Aliotta et al. 2008). Despite the increasing attention that is paid to family caregivers, empirical evidence suggests that there are large unmet training needs. Training is rarely provided for current caregiving tasks and anticipated future caregiving responsibilities (Wilkins, Bruce and Sirey 2009). Moreover, there are clear context- and culture-specific limits to what family caregivers can do for patients with chronic diseases (Levine 1999).

New settings

Single-handed practices are no longer seen as the role model for medicine. The trend internationally is moving towards **group practices** that are more patient oriented and more cost-effective (Busse and Schlette 2003). In Canada, for example, a major part of the health reform involves developing models in which doctors work within a team with nurses, social workers, psychologists, dieticians, midwives and physiotherapists. The aim is to create a primary health care system more closely oriented to the needs of the patients: multidisciplinary, well coordinated and accessible 24 hours a day (Torgerson 2005a). In Germany, polyclinics with general practitioners (GPs), specialists and other health professionals were reintroduced in 2004 (Busse, Zentner and Schlette 2006).

In many countries in which strong primary care teams already exist, such as the United Kingdom, the Netherlands and Scandinavia, the management of many chronic diseases has been moving progressively to **nurse-led clinics** (Nolte and McKee 2008; Buchan and Calman 2005). These clinics have become more common in managing diabetes and hypertension, allergy/asthma/COPD, psychiatry and heart failure (Karlberg 2008). The main reasons for this growth are economic in nature, as well as the chance to create new career opportunities for nurses. Other developments improve access through telephone consultations and offer support for elderly individuals with communication difficulties.

4.3 Coordinating care for individual chronic diseases: DMPs

This section examines care models for individual chronic diseases, and the following section analyses integrated care approaches. DMPs are normally limited to health care workers, while concepts of integrated care often include social workers. However, the concepts of **integrated care** and **disease management** are in some respects similar.

There are several definitions of DMPs, but most share three main features: a knowledge base, a delivery system with coordinated care, and a continuous improvement process for a specific disease within a specific population (Hunter and Fairfield 1997). Key elements are shown in Box 4.1.

Box 4.1 *Disease management: key elements*

- Comprehensive care: multidisciplinary care for entire disease cycle
- Integrated care, care continuum, coordination of the different components
- Population orientation (defined by a specific condition)
- Active client–patient management tools (health education, empowerment, self-care)
- Evidence-based guidelines, protocols, care pathways
- Information technology, system solutions
- Continuous quality improvement

Source: Velasco-Garrido, Busse and Hisashige 2003.

To summarize, disease management is a means of coordinating care that focuses on the entire clinical course of a disease. Care is organized and delivered according to scientific evidence and patients are actively involved.

Structured DMPs for selected conditions were originally developed in the United States, then in a range of European countries. This approach seems promising, particularly when health care is funded through social insurance. Because these systems tend to allow patients to choose family practitioners and some specialists, doctors are more likely to work as single-handed practitioners. This leads to a separation between the ambulatory and hospital sectors, and DMPs could overcome this (Nolte and McKee 2008).

In 2002 in Germany, for example, programmes were introduced that now cover diabetes types 1 and 2, asthma/COPD, coronary heart disease and breast cancer.

In December 2006 there were 10 580 programmes with nearly 2.7 million patients (BVA 2008). By April 2008, this number had risen to 4.7 million (Van Lente, Willenborg and Egger 2008). Table 4.2 provides a breakdown of those DMPs.

Table 4.2 *DMP participants in Germany according to indication (2008)*

DMP	Number of patients enrolled in DMP
Diabetes mellitus type 2	2 708 154
Diabetes mellitus type 1	93 357
Coronary heart disease	1 221 374
Asthma	313 914
COPD	264 299
Breast cancer	100 499
Total	*4 701 597*

Source: Van Lente, Willenborg and Egger 2008.

Until the end of 2008, risk structure compensation schemes took DMPs into account by calculating expenditure for these patients separately. This created strong incentives for sickness funds to enrol patients. They also provided sizeable financial incentives for the doctors taking part (Busse 2004). Since January 2009, participation in DMPs alone is no longer taken into account as a separate risk-adjustment factor. Instead, the allocation formula provides supplements for individuals suffering from one of 80 (mainly chronic) diseases. For every insured person classified as suffering from one (or several) of these conditions, the sickness funds receive an extra allocation. Hence, for the first time a detailed measure of morbidity is being used to assess risk, superseding in some way the use of DMPs as a risk-adjustment tool. Sickness funds no longer receive separate funding for those enrolled in DMPs. The new system removes the financial incentive to run DMPs, a strong driver for the establishment of these programmes from 2004 until 2008. As a consequence, since 2009, DMPs have to prove to be attractive and cost-effective in their own right in order to survive. Moreover, as classification is partly based on medication, a problem could arise, in that insurers may try to benefit from extra funding by motivating providers to prescribe certain medications, irrespective of disease severity (Schang 2009).

Sweden now has **chains of care** (Andersson and Karlberg 2000), defined as "coordinated activities within health care", often involving "several responsible authorities and medical providers" (Åhgren 2003). County councils are responsible for organizing health care and by 2002 most of them had at least one chain of care, mostly designed around patients with diabetes, dementia and rheumatoid disorders (Nolte and McKee 2008).

4.4 Managing care across chronic diseases: integrated care models

DMPs focusing on a single disease have increasingly come under pressure. Doctors and researchers admit they have focused on a straightforward disease management approach because it was relatively simple. However, chronic conditions do not present alone, so various countries are experimenting with new models of health care delivery – comprehensive **integrated care models** or **provider networks** that can achieve more integrated and more comprehensive services.

Integrated care models developed in the United States have been influential in Europe (Nolte and McKee 2008). The redesign of health care services has been guided by approaches taken by the United States health maintenance organization Kaiser Permanente (Goodwin et al. 2004), the Evercare model developed by UnitedHealth Group (UnitedHealth Europe 2005) and the **Chronic Care Model** (CCM) developed by Edward Wagner (Wagner et al. 1999).

These have been used as the basis for United Kingdom NHS programmes since 2003 (Nolte and McKee 2008). The Evercare model of managing frail elderly people was piloted in nine PCTs in April 2003, and case management then became part of the Government's policy for supporting people with chronic conditions. The 2004 NHS Improvement Plan stipulated the introduction of case management in all PCTs by appointing senior nurses (known as **community matrons**) by 2007 (Department of Health 2004).

In 2005 the United Kingdom launched a model designed to help health and social care organizations improve care for people with chronic conditions (Singh and Fahey 2008). It built on United States approaches, such as the CCM, the Kaiser Triangle and the Evercare model (Department of Health 2004). It outlined how people with chronic conditions were to be identified and receive care according to their needs. The goals of the NHS and social care model are to improve the quality and accessibility of care for people with chronic conditions and to contain or reduce the associated costs (Singh and Fahey 2008).

Various autonomous communes in Spain have been operating pilot projects on the long-term integration of care for many years. These aim to achieve complete health care by providing complete care from one source only and by implementing regional strategies. For example, the Spanish region of Valencia has been testing local, population-based integration models in three areas since 1997 (Campoy 2005).

In Germany, various models have been introduced to promote more integrated care, such as DMPs (see Section 4.3), care models based on the family physician as gatekeeper, integrated care contracts, and medical polyclinics. The integrated care contracts include at least two entities from different health care sectors or interdisciplinary collaborations. Between 2004 and 2008, 1% of the total payments for physicians and hospitals was earmarked for investment into integrated care projects. This involved re-allocating approximately €680 million per year. There has been – and still is – a remarkable variety of contracts. For example, most of them are related to a specific indication, such as stroke, or to a specific medical procedure, such as hip replacement. Population-based approaches are rarely taken (Busse, Zentner and Schlette 2006). Recently, analysts recommended the CCM as a means of advancing the countrywide approach started in 2002 (Beyer et al. 2006).

Various provider networks have been developed in Europe and elsewhere. In France the 1996 Juppé reforms introduced mechanisms aimed at stimulating local provider networks for ambulatory patients and at improving the interface between ambulatory and hospital care (Bras, Duhamel and Grass 2006; Sandier, Paris and Polton 2004). Initiatives were formalized in 2002 under the heading of **health networks** *(réseaux de santé)* (Frossard et al. 2002). These arrangements now include mobile dialysis units, specialized mental health care facilities, new cancer centres (combining research, treatment and prevention) and new centres for managing HIV/AIDS (McKee and Healy 2002).

The Netherlands has also been trying to improve the continuity and quality of care for people with long-term conditions and to close the gap between primary and hospital services. This led to the concept of **transmural care** in the early 1990s (Van der Linden, Spreeuwenberg and Schrijvers 2001), which has since been developed extensively, with an estimated total of over 500 initiatives in place by 1999 (Van der Linden, Spreeuwenberg and Schrijvers 2001). Most forms of transmural care tend to focus on those who are not able to return to a fully independent life by managing the interface between acute hospital care and alternative settings (Nolte and McKee 2008).

The Canadian province of Ontario has chosen to promote networks of family doctors (family health groups and family health networks) and local health integration networks. The mission of these local care networks is to improve the planning, coordination and integration of health care. Being local organizations, they are expected to be more responsive to local needs (Torgerson 2005b).

Chapter 5
Effectiveness of strategies against chronic disease

Evaluating a health programme requires looking at health improvement as measured, for example, by patients' quantity and/or quality of life. This chapter examines the available evidence on various strategies and interventions.

5.1 Prevention and early detection

Studies have looked at a range of interventions. Measures to reduce tobacco consumption have been analysed in considerable depth (see Section 4.1). Effective interventions include higher prices for cigarettes, public smoking bans, public information, bans on advertising and promotion, smoking cessation programmes and smuggling controls (Table 5.1). Combining various measures is more effective than individual measures. Anti-tobacco regulations therefore should be as comprehensive as possible and combine a number of different mechanisms (Busse and Schlette 2007).

Opposition to measures such as smoking bans has come from vested interests and public opinion. Increasingly more countries – such as Ireland, Italy, Malta, New Zealand, Norway, Singapore and Sweden – have introduced a complete ban on smoking in public places and at work. Similar regulations have been introduced in other countries, including Australia, the Czech Republic, England, Finland, Germany, Hungary, Portugal, Scotland and Spain. However, public support varies considerably. The first countries introduced rigid bans some years ago and, after initial scepticism, people have increasingly come to accept them (Busse and Schlette 2007).

Diet can be affected substantially by changing production processes to reduce unhealthy components of food, such as trans-fat or salt. These changes can be implemented quickly if the private sector and/or governments are supportive.

Table 5.1 *Effects of antismoking measures on smoker prevalence*

Measure	Effect on smoker prevalence
Price increase by 10%	Decline by 4 percentage points in countries with high per capita income
Ban on smoking at work	Decline by 5–10 percentage points
Bans on smoking in pubs, restaurants and other public places	Decline by 2–4 percentage points
Advertising ban	Decline by 6 percentage points if ban is absolute
Health warning on cigarette packs	In the Netherlands, 28% of all 13- to 18-year-olds said they smoked less as a result of the health warnings
	In Belgium, 8% of those asked said they smoked less because of warnings
Media campaigns	Percentage of smokers declines by 5–10 percentage points, depending on how the campaigns are targeted at specific groups
Withdrawal measures; subsidies for treatment	Decline by 1–2 percentage points after 2 years, depending on the people registered

Source: European Network for Smoking Prevention 2004.

For example, government-induced changes in manufacturing processes in Mauritius and Poland appear to have reduced risk factors for chronic diseases (Zatonski, McMichael and Powles 1998).

There is clear evidence that anti-hypertensive and anti-cholesterol medications, as well as aspirin, reduce the risk of ischaemic heart disease and stroke (Rodgers et al. 2006). A combination of education, careful monitoring according to clinical guidelines, and fixed dose therapies improves patient adherence, which is notoriously hard to do (Novotny 2008).

Overall, prevention still plays a secondary role in most health systems and few countries have set up programmes to prevent chronic diseases.

5.2 New provider qualifications and settings

Primary care nurses with enhanced roles can provide high-quality care in many areas traditionally within the domain of family doctors (Dubois, Singh and Jiwani 2008). But most studies have included only small numbers of clinicians and have not examined long-term outcomes (Brown and Grimes 1995; Horrocks, Anderson and Salisbury 2002). It has long been established that the availability of specialist nurses for care of patients with long-term conditions may improve health outcomes and reduce use of health resources (Boaden et al. 2006; Griffiths, Foster and Barnes 2004; Singh 2005a; Smith, Bury and O'Leary 2004). Some researchers have questioned this, suggesting that nurse practitioners may reduce hospital admissions, but at the same time introducing more services into primary care (Sargent et al. 2007). Furthermore, preliminary evidence suggests that benefits from case management in terms of health and financial outcomes are hard to trace (Gravelle et al. 2007).

Clinics run by specialist nurses have been associated with better clinical outcomes (Connor, Wright and Fegan 2002; Singh 2005b; Vrijhoef, Diederiks and Spreeuwenberg 2000; Vrijhoef et al. 2001; Vrijhoef et al. 2003). Patient satisfaction with nurse-led care is generally high (Horrocks, Anderson and Salisbury 2002; Kinnersley, Anderson and Parry 2000; Shum, Humphreys and Wheeler 2000). Research in Sweden, for example, showed that nurse-led heart failure clinics – giving education, better treatment and social support – improved survival and self-care behaviour, and reduced the need for hospital care (Cline 2002; Stromberg, Martensson and Fridlund 2003). However, the precise effect was hard to identify because their implementation was part of an overall reorganization of care (Dubois, Singh and Jiwani 2008).

Moreover, it has been shown that perceived caregiving competence and practical support by health professionals are associated with optimum family caregiving (Greenberger and Litwin 2003). This suggests that providing support, training and qualifications to family caregivers can represent effective strategies for tackling chronic conditions (Wilkins, Bruce and Sirey 2009).

5.3 Coordinating care for individual chronic diseases: DMPs

Evidence on the effectiveness of DMPs comes from several systematic reviews and meta-reviews.

In 2002 a meta-review of 118 DMPs examined the effectiveness of different strategies in chronic disease management (Weingarten, Henning and Badamgarav 2002). Those using provider education, feedback and/or reminders produced better adherence by providers to care guidelines. However, the meta-review did not show which approaches produced the greatest relative improvement, as the studies did not directly compare different approaches. The authors concluded that it was not possible to prepare policy recommendations on developing DMPs.

Another study concluded that appropriately evaluated DMPs improved the quality of care as measured by the provider's increased adherence to evidence-based standards and by disease control (Velasco Garrido, Busse and Hisashige 2003). However, evidence of the effectiveness of the programmes was found only for diabetes, depression, coronary heart disease and heart failure (McAlister et al. 2001a; McAlister et al. 2001b; Weingarten, Henning and Badamgarav 2002; Norris et al. 2002). For other chronic conditions the results were inconclusive. Effectiveness referred only to process and structure, and no study found any statistically significant impact on (long-term) health outcomes.

The findings on patients' quality of life and on patients' and providers' satisfaction were also inconclusive.

A related study (Ofman, Badamgarav and Henning 2004) found that improvements in quality of care (as measured by patient satisfaction) were greatest with treatment, patient adherence to treatment recommendations, and measures of disease control. Nolte and McKee (2008) suggest that disease management may be an effective method of changing the behaviour of patients and providers.

A recent meta-review (Mattke, Seid and Sai 2007) concluded that DMPs improve processes of care and disease control. However, the authors found no evidence of any effect on health outcomes. Disease management did not seem to affect utilization, except for reducing hospitalization rates among patients with congestive heart failure (CHF), and increasing outpatient care and prescription drug use among patients with depression (Mattke, Seid and Sai 2007).

These are preliminary findings, because most of the empirical work looked at small-scale programmes run for high-risk individuals as demonstration projects on a single site. These pilot projects mostly combined individual patient education, care planning, and follow-up delivered by a nurse or case manager. Such levels of support would be difficult to maintain in large-scale DMPs.

Most evidence exists for CHF and diabetes mellitus, with CHF standing out in particular. Sufficient research was also identified for coronary artery disease (CAD), asthma, COPD and depression, but not for other chronic conditions such as cancer, dementia, Alzheimer's disease and musculoskeletal disorders (Table 5.2).

Generally, the evidence suggests that DMPs can improve the care process. Improvements in clinical care affect intermediate outcomes and disease control for CHF, CAD, diabetes mellitus and depression. The impact of these programmes on long-term outcomes has not yet been established, so it is impossible to draw any general conclusions.

The evidence relating to the impact of DMPs on utilization of health services is generally inconclusive. A few studies compare patients taking part in programmes with those following "normal" care paths. These were found to reduce hospitalization rates for those with CHF, but increase use of outpatient care and prescription drugs.

Table 5.2 Summary of evidence for various disease management programme outcomes, by disease

Disease	Clinical processes Adherence to evidence-based guidelines	Health-related Changes in behaviours	Disease control Changes in intermediate measures	Clinical outcomes	Health care utilization Changes in utilization of services	Financial outcomes	Patient experience Satisfaction, quality of life, etc.
CHF	Improved	Inconclusive evidence	Improved	Inconclusive evidence	Reduced hospital admission rates	Inconclusive evidence	Improved
CAD	Improved	Evidence for no effect	Improved	Evidence for no effect	Inconclusive evidence	Inconclusive evidence	Insufficient evidence
Diabetes	Improved	Evidence for no effect	Improved	Insufficient evidence	Inconclusive evidence	Inconclusive evidence	Insufficient evidence
Asthma	Inconclusive evidence	Inconclusive evidence	Inconclusive evidence	Evidence for no effect	Inconclusive evidence	Evidence for no effect	Insufficient evidence
COPD	Insufficient evidence	Insufficient evidence	Inconclusive evidence	Insufficient evidence	Insufficient evidence	Insufficient evidence	Insufficient evidence
Depression	Improved	n/a	Improved	Inconclusive evidence	Increased utilization	Increased costs	Improved

Source: Mattke, Seid and Sai 2007.

Note: n/a: Not available.

Overall, the evidence on DMPs is far from satisfactory, given its prominent role. Few studies have looked at the effects of large-scale population-based interventions (Table 5.3).

Table 5.3 *Findings from studies of large-scale, population-based disease management programmes*

Author	Setting	Managed condition(s)	Comparison strategy	Results
Sidorov et al. (2002)	Programme developed and operated by integrated delivery system	Diabetes	Programme participants versus non-participants, controlled for age, sex, insurance type, duration of plan enrolment, presence of improved use of pharmaceuticals	Improved quality of care and disease control, lower costs and utilization, net costs saving
Fireman, Bartlett and Selby (2004)	Programme developed and operated by integrated delivery system	CAD, CHF, diabetes, asthma	Patients with the condition versus those without, matched by age and sex	Improved quality of care and disease control, costs increased less in intervention group than in reference group, no net cost saving
Villagra and Ahmed (2004)	Programme developed and operated by disease management vendor for health plan client	Diabetes	Natural experiment created by phased roll-out, plus pre–post comparison, adjustment for risk and demographic differences	Improved quality of care, lower cost and utilization in both comparisons, net cost savings

Source: Mattke, Seid and Sai 2007.

What studies there are conclude that population-based interventions improve patient care. The results must be interpreted carefully, however, because none of the studies was randomized, and only one used a rigorous comparison. The evidence relating to cost is also inconclusive. Sidorov and colleagues (2002), as well as Villagra and Ahmed (2004) found net cost savings for DMPs, but Fireman and colleagues examined four chronic conditions and did not find net cost savings.

Unfortunately, in Germany a unique opportunity to evaluate DMPs on a large scale has been missed. While evaluation of DMPs is mandatory – and includes the fulfilment of medical parameters, the observation of rules of enrollment for and costs of services – it is conceived methodologically as an uncontrolled, post-intervention only, prospective cohort study; basically, the weakest design possible (Blümel and Busse 2009).

One study which used a 3-armed prospective cluster-randomized design was the German ELSID-Diabetes study (Evaluation of a Large-Scale Implementation of Disease Management Programs), set up in 2005 to assess the effectiveness of a diabetes DMP in primary care within two German federal states (Joos, Rosemann and Heiderhoff 2005). Early results show that the death rate among patients in the programme dropped significantly (10.9%) over two and a half years compared with those receiving "standard" care (18.8%). Age-adjusted evaluations among severely ill women showed a significant variation: 9.5% of those on the programme compared with 12.3% of others (Szecsenyi et al. 2008). The data for men are not yet available. The study also found that patients taking part in a programme perceived their care as more structured and coordinated than did those receiving standard care (Szecsenyi 2008).

Recently, Ose and colleagues (2009) examined the effectiveness of the German diabetes DMPs based on the ELSID data for patients with varying numbers of other medical conditions with respect to their health-related quality of life (HRQoL). The EQ-5D score, a standardized measure of health outcomes used to draw conclusions on HRQoL, was analysed by grouping patients according to those inscribed into a DMP and those receiving routine chronic care. Their analysis suggests that participation in the DMP ($p<0.001$), the number of other conditions ($p<0.001$) and the interaction between the DMP and the number of other conditions ($p<0.05$) had a significant impact on the EQ-5D score. They conclude that the number of other conditions may have a negative impact on the HRQoL and that the German DMP for type 2 diabetes may help to counterbalance this effect.

Despite these results, overall there is a lack of systematic evaluations of population-based chronic DMPs in Europe. This is partly because DMPs have been introduced relatively recently (Nolte and McKee 2008). Their impact depends heavily on their context, so research from high-income countries outside Europe are of limited value.

5.4 Managing care across chronic diseases: integrated care models

The evidence on different models of integrated care is inconclusive (Nolte and McKee 2008). Studies have found that one or more components of the CCM benefits some processes and outcomes, but the evidence does not show whether the whole model is needed to achieve the same benefits (Singh and Ham 2006).

One analysis looked at the effectiveness of the six components of the CCM, focusing particularly on primary care (Table 5.4) (Zwar et al. 2006). From a systematic review, along with a review of reviews, the authors identified a series of effective key elements and approaches.

Table 5.4 *Summary of evidence on effectiveness of CCM components*

CCM component	Interventions shown to be effective	Outcome measures affected

Patient self-management support	• Patient educational sessions
	• Patient motivational counselling
	• Distribution of educational materials
		• Physiological measures of disease
		• Patient
		  • quality of life
		  • health status
		  • functional status
		  • satisfaction with service
		  • risk behaviour
		  • knowledge
		  • service use
		  • adherence to treatment

Delivery system design	• Multidisciplinary teams	• Physiological measures of disease • Professionals' adherence to guidelines • Patient service use
Decision support	• Implementation of evidence-based guidelines • Educational meetings with professionals • Distribution of educational materials among professionals	• Professionals' adherence to guidelines • Physiological measures of disease
Clinical information systems	• Audit and feedback	• Professionals' adherence to guidelines
Delivery system	Little published experimental evidence	
Community resources	Little published experimental evidence	

Source: Zwar et al. 2006; Nolte and McKee 2008.

Components influencing adherence to guidelines were found to include self-management support and delivery system design, particularly when combined with decision support and clinical information systems.

However, Zwar and colleagues' conclusions must be treated with caution. The findings are based on the management of adults with type 2 diabetes and may not be transferable to other chronic conditions or other age groups. It is also unclear whether broader components of the CCM – such as health care organization and/or community resources – have caused the changes. It is difficult to examine the effect of this model in experimental studies, which may explain why such studies are rare (Zwar et al. 2006).

Piatt and colleagues (2006) found preliminary evidence relating to the CCM as a whole. In an experimental study, they examined the effect on clinical and behavioural outcomes of patients with diabetes. They targeted small practices in an underserved area of Pittsburgh in the United States. Substantial improvements were found after 12 months for two clinical outcomes and for self-monitoring of blood glucose in the CCM group compared with control groups (provider intervention; standard care). Otherwise no statistically significant outcomes were found.

Another United States study examined the impact of the CCM approach on the quality of care for patients with diabetes, coronary heart disease and depression (Solberg et al. 2006). After two years the organization had adopted most elements of the CCM, and the quality of care for patients with diabetes and coronary heart disease had improved. Nevertheless, no significant correlation could be established between these changes.

Self-management support and delivery systems – identified in other studies as the most important CCM elements (Singh 2005a; Zwar et al. 2006) – did not bring about significant improvements. Evidence of the effectiveness of the CCM is not overwhelming, but this may be because the model is not being implemented properly. One qualitative study examined potential barriers during the implementation process (Hroscikoski et al. 2006). They found too many competing priorities, plus a lack of specificity of changes, agreement about the care process, and engagement by health professionals (especially doctors). The authors concluded that the CCM is useful as a conceptual framework, but should be supplemented by guidelines on implementation.

There is also limited evidence on the impact of provider networks. Studies in France have suggested rather positive effects, with fewer drug prescriptions, fewer hospitalizations and lower mortality rates (Singh 2008).

A study in Canada also recently examined provider networks – an ambulatory care centre with a group practice and multidisciplinary teams using electronic medical records. The study looked at nine process outcomes and three clinical outcomes: blood pressure, HbA1c levels and lipids. The results suggest positive outcomes, especially for blood pressure targets and HbA1c outcomes (Suhrcke, Fahey and McKee 2008).

Chapter 6

Cost–effectiveness of strategies against chronic disease

Although different instruments and approaches have been developed to tackle chronic diseases, resources are limited. Policy-makers have to prioritize between different strategies. Cost–effectiveness analysis determines how much health improvement is gained for each monetary unit spent and is a systematic and sophisticated tool for deciding on priorities. However, cost–effectiveness analysis demands considerable data, which means that many management strategies lack sophisticated evaluations, particularly in Europe. There are also many methodological problems, and it can be difficult to establish whether a specific programme or component is effective from a health perspective. Furthermore, it is not always easy to measure the costs of conducting a specific programme. This chapter summarizes the available evidence on cost–effectiveness.

6.1 Prevention and early detection

Cost–effectiveness studies have found that individual and group approaches to chronic disease prevention may be highly cost-effective. However, the success of interventions is largely determined by regional differences in cost structures and in the burden of chronic diseases.

For tobacco control, the World Bank (Jha and Chaloupka 2000) and the Disease Control Priorities Project (2007) have found evidence indicating cost-effectiveness; this is not surprising considering the health benefits. The main intervention targeted at individuals is over-the-counter nicotine-replacement therapy. These strategies have been applied successfully and are cost-effective (Jha et al. 2006).

The evidence relating to interventions to prevent or reduce obesity (and consequently diabetes) is inconclusive. Cawley (2007) identified costs for primary, secondary and tertiary preventions ranging from US$4305 for school-based interventions to US$35 600 for bariatric surgery, using quality-adjusted life years (QALYs) saved as an end-point (Table 6.1).

Table 6.1 *Cost per QALY saved by interventions to reduce or prevent obesity*

Intervention	Target population	Estimated cost per QALY (US$)	Source
Planet health (a school-based intervention to improve nutrition and increase physical activity)	Middle-school children	Girls: 4 305	Wang et al. (2003)
Orlistat[a]	Overweight and obese patients with type 2 diabetes mellitus	8 327	Maetzel et al. (2003)
Bariatric surgery	Middle-aged men and women who are morbidly obese	Women: 5400–16 100 Men: 10 000–35 600	Craig and Tseng (2002)
Diet, exercise, and behaviour modification	Adult women	12 640	Roux et al. (2006)

Source: Cawley 2007.
[a] Pharmaceutical intervention to reduce adiposities.

Another study found that "self-management diabetes education", physical activity and diet were cost-effective for preventing diabetes (Narayan Venkat et al. 2006). Given the dependence of such strategies upon context, cost–effectiveness is likely to vary according to regional settings. Parallel interventions at social, health system, and individual levels would seem to be needed in order to prevent the rise of obesity and diabetes throughout Europe.

Screening for greater risk of cardiovascular disease is cost-effective, according to the evidence. However, the number of proven screening procedures for chronic diseases is limited (Novotny 2008).

Results differ for primary prevention of cardiovascular disease. Controlling blood pressure with drugs or serum cholesterol is highly cost-effective for those with risk factors, and sometimes cost-effective for the general population. But there are marked differences.

For high-risk adults over 45 years with high blood pressure (over 105 mmHg diastolic pressure), drug treatment may only cost a few hundred dollars per life year gained. On average across all age groups, however, drug treatment costs

US$4600 to US$100 000 per life year gained. Differences in underlying risks, age and cost of medication explain the enormous difference in cost–effectiveness (Rodgers et al. 2006).

Cost–effectiveness ratios for cholesterol-lowering interventions are improving, but they vary significantly by age and risk level. Some evidence has suggested that dietary interventions for reducing cholesterol can also be cost-effective, costing about US$2000 per QALY (Prosser et al. 2000).

6.2 New provider qualifications and settings

So far there is no conclusive evidence on the cost–effectiveness of new qualifications, such as those for nurse practitioners or case managers.

Studies increasingly confirm that nurse-led clinics result in better health outcomes (Nolte and McKee 2008) and often also lead to better compliance (Vrijhoef et al. 2001; Singh 2005b). There is some evidence for this, but it is not possible to generalize on the findings (Smith et al. 2001).

6.3 Coordinating care for individual chronic diseases: DMPs

The original goal of DMPs when first introduced in the United States was to reduce costs (Pilnick, Dingwall and Starkey 2001). It was expected that using the programmes to change usage would lower hospitalization and complication rates and be more efficient.

However, few studies included measures of utilization, such as emergency department visits or hospitalizations. Economic evaluations of DMPs tend to focus only on costs, while benefits and cost-benefits are rarely considered (Velasco-Garrido, Busse and Hisashige 2003; Ofman, Badamgarav and Henning 2004). Ofman and colleagues, along with Velasco-Garrido and colleagues conclude that there is no evidence that DMPs are more cost-effective than standard care.

Mattke and colleagues (Mattke, Seid and Sai 2007) draw similar conclusions. Their comprehensive review found that many studies have methodological flaws, such as incomplete accounting for costs or a lack of a suitable control group. Even looking at the reported costs and the savings generated rarely brings to light any conclusive evidence that disease management brings about net savings on direct medical costs.

Furthermore, the long-term and medium-term impact of DMPs has not yet been studied satisfactorily. As a consequence, no conclusions can be drawn about the financial returns on investment (Nolte and McKee 2008).

6.4 Managing care across chronic diseases: integrated care models

The economic impact of integrated care models in Europe has not yet been studied in full. There is some evidence on the Evercare approach to case management. United States-based studies have found that it is cheaper to care for older people in nursing homes (Nolte and McKee 2008). The main reason for this is the related, more appropriate use of resources, especially hospitals and emergency services (Kane et al. 2004; UnitedHealth Europe 2005). However, evaluations of the Evercare pilot in England did not find improvements such as lower emergency admissions and fewer bed days (Gravelle et al. 2007).

Bodenheimer and colleauges (Bodenheimer, Wagner and Grumbach 2002b) carried out a review-of-reviews on the CCM and its impact on use of resources and costs in terms of CHF, asthma and diabetes. They reviewed 27 studiesand found that backing for self-management support was the most common component, followed by delivery system redesign (such as the introduction of follow-up by means of home visits, multispecialty teams, nurse-led clinics and case management – mostly for CHF and diabetes). The findings were mixed. Some approaches showed positive results (for example, fewer hospital admissions or visits to emergency departments, and/or cost reductions), but others did not. This means that no general conclusions can be drawn, especially since there was a lack of population-based interventions, context-specific variables were not controlled and sophisticated comparison with other strategies in chronic disease management was largely absent (Nolte and McKee 2008).

Part III
Challenges of chronic disease management

Based on the evidence presented in Chapters 4–6, this part outlines and discusses five institutional and organizational challenges that policy-makers need to consider in order to tackle chronic disease successfully:

1. *stimulating the development of new, effective pharmaceuticals and medical devices*

2. *designing appropriate financial incentives*

3. *improving coordination and cooperation*

4. *using information and communication techhnology*

5. *ensuring evaluation.*

Chapter 7
Tackling the challenges of chronic disease in Europe

Tackling chronic disease in Europe successfully will be a challenge. The epidemiologic and economic analyses suggest that policy-makers should make disease management a top priority. However, choosing the right strategies will be difficult, particularly given the limited evidence on effectiveness and cost–effectiveness. Policy-makers need more than academic evidence on individual interventions; they also need to know which institutional and organizational conditions favour successful chronic disease management and where the gaps in knowledge need to be reduced. This chapter gives policy-makers the relevant insights for effectively tackling chronic disease and suggests areas of research that will help them to draw further conclusions.

7.1 New pharmaceuticals and medical devices

Pharmaceuticals and medical devices are essential for diagnosis and treatment. Many licensed drugs – such as anti-hypertensives, insulin, antidepressants, anti-inflammatories and inhaled steroids – target chronic diseases. These treatments have become increasingly sophisticated, sometimes targeting elements of the disease process that were unknown at the end of the 1980s.

Despite the important role of pharmaceuticals, the debate on chronic disease management tends to concentrate on structures and programmes. The following subsection looks at new pharmaceutical approaches. Reviewing drug development for individual diseases is beyond the scope of this book: rather, it will examine broad trends and highlight some advances.

Improvement in compliance

Successfully managing chronic disease requires not only effective drugs but also effective and sustained self-management, such as medication compliance (Bangalore et al. 2007). Compliance, or adherence, can be defined as the extent to which patients follow medical instructions (WHO 2003). In 2003 the WHO report *Adherence to long-term therapies* found that compliance by patients with long-term diseases – such as cardiovascular diseases or depression – was poor. Only about 50% of patients in developed countries adhered to their treatment: in the United States, for example, the proportion of patients adhering to their high blood pressure regimen was 51%. Similar patterns were reported for other conditions such as depression (40%) and asthma (43% for acute treatments and 28% for maintenance) (WHO 2003).

Many factors affect adherence. Most notable are those related to the complexity of the medical regimen, length of treatment, previous treatment failures, frequent changes in treatment, the immediacy of beneficial effects, and side-effects and the availability of medical support to deal with them (WHO 2003; Bloom 2001). A systematic review (Van Dulmen et al. 2007) outlined various methods of improving adherence, as detailed here.

- *Technical interventions:* simpler medication regimens, for example, dosage, packaging or combining drugs.

- *Behavioural interventions:* memory aids and reminders, for example, by mail, telephone, computer or home visits.

- *Educational interventions:* teaching and providing knowledge through individual and group education, face-to-face contact and audio-visual techniques.

- *Social support interventions:* practical and emotional support by family, friends and health professionals.

- *Structural interventions:* DMPs and community care.

- *Complex or multifaceted interventions:* combining and adopting different approaches and interventions.

Research into pharmaceuticals and medical devices now recognizes the importance of technical interventions that could increase adherence. For example, one meta-review (Bangalore et al. 2007) concluded that fixed-dose combinations can improve compliance by reducing the pill burden (polypharmacy). Fixed-dose combinations also reduced the risk of noncompliance by 24%. Wald and Law (2003) proposed the use of a "polypill" that would include a statin with three anti-hypertensive medications – a thiazide, a beta-blocker and an angiotensin-converting enzyme inhibitor – in addition to folic acid and aspirin. They estimated that if everyone over 55 years of age with pre-existing CAD took this one pill, the risk of ischaemic heart disease could be reduced by 88% and the risk of stroke by 80%. Whether this "magic bullet" is practical or not is open to debate, but these two studies show that compliance and health outcomes can be improved by fixed-drug combinations.

Simplifying the medication regimen also seems to increase compliance. A meta-analysis (Claxton, Cramer and Pierce 2001) concluded that 79% (±14%) of patients took "once daily" doses, 65% (±15%) "three times daily" and only 51% (±20%) "four times daily".

Quality of life in pharmaceutical care

Improvement of adherence is closely linked to the concept of quality of life. In 1948, WHO defined health as a "state of complete physical, mental and social well-being and not merely the absence of disease or infirmity" (WHO 1991). This broadened the concept of health beyond the biomedical model. Today, pharmaceuticals are intended to improve the patient's quality of life as well as achieve better clinical outcomes; this is important with chronic conditions, for which there is often no cure. Pharmaceuticals for most chronic diseases aim to prevent and control symptoms, reduce the frequency and severity of exacerbations and improve general health. A better quality of life is their more realistic objective (Kheir et al. 2004).

The chronically ill are often restricted in their daily lives, with phases of poor functional, mental and social skills. The burden of diagnosis and treatment can be high (for instance, chemotherapy and radiotherapy in cancer treatment) and can be accompanied by psychosocial implications, such as those affecting social involvement, partnership and workforce, along with stigma and pain (Petermann 1996). "Supportive" drugs that improve the quality of life become more important. They are less toxic, often administered orally, and enable patients to spend fewer days in hospital (Wilking and Jönsson 2005).

Taking this into consideration, the assessment of pharmaceuticals in chronic care has to go beyond considering whether the patient has been cured or not. It seems more appropriate to be using quality of life as a key criterion for chronic disease management, but to use this concept for decisions on approval, therapy and reimbursement requires valid and objective methods of evaluation.

Personalized medicine

Developments in drug therapy aim for a good response with easy application, fixed doses and mild side-effects. The different ways in which patients respond is determined by personal factors (such as genetics, age, gender, other disease and/or drug therapy and environmental agents) and by drug factors (such as pharmacokinetics, pharmacodynamics, adverse effects and drug interactions). Personalized medicine aims to optimize drug therapy in the face of these factors (Lewis 2005). Advances in human genome research have replaced the linear process of drug discovery and development by an integrated and heuristic approach (Ginsburg and McCarthy 2001). Table 7.1 gives some examples.

Table 7.1 *Personalized medicine*

Drug	Disease(s) or condition(s) treated
Abatacept	Rheumatoid arthritis
Adalimumab	Crohn's disease, psoriatic arthritis, rheumatoid arthritis
Anakinra	Rheumatoid arthritis
Efalizumab	Psoriasis
Epoprostenol sodium	Primary pulmonary hypertension
Etanercept	Ankylosing spondylitis, juvenile rheumatoid arthritis, psoriatic arthritis, rheumatoid arthritis
Glatiramer	Multiple sclerosis
Imiglucerase	Gaucher's disease
Infliximab	Ankylosing spondylitis, Crohn's disease, psoriasis, psoriatic arthritis, rheumatoid arthritis, ulcerative colitis
Interferon beta-1a	Multiple sclerosis
Interferon beta-1b	Multiple sclerosis
Laronidase	Hurler's disease
Natalizumab	Multiple sclerosis
Omalizumab	Asthma
Palivizumab	Respiratory syncytial virus
Peginterferon alfa-2b	Hepatitis C
Peginterferon alfa-2a	Hepatitis C
Treporstinil sodium	Primary pulmonary hypertension

Source: Shane 2007.

Cancer research, for example, is now using pharmacogenomics to personalize drug therapy. Advances in genetics are used to explain individual differences in drug responses (Shurin and Nabel 2008). The advances in molecular medicine mean that traditional anti-tumour agents have been replaced by new agents with milder side-effects that target disease-specific mechanisms. Gene/protein expression analyses make treatment more accurate as well as improving imaging techniques. Cancer researchers are working on deciphering the human proteome, which has considerable potential. The main areas in which new agents have been developed and are now used in clinical practice are as follows (Wilking and Jönsson 2005):

- targeting the cell cycle apoptosis

- replicating/transcripting and repairing DNA

- inhibiting hormones, growth factors and cell signalling pathways

- inhibiting new blood vessels (angiogenesis).

Cancer research illustrates that personalized medicine is an important factor in developing innovative pharmaceuticals for the chronically ill. Apart from increasing cures, it may lead to drugs that improve the patient's quality of life.

Policy recommendations

- Personalized drugs are one of the main trends in the development of pharmaceuticals. However, using specialized medication to manage chronic disease brings about a new set of problems. In particular, policy-makers at government level, in regulatory authorities as well as those responsible for the payer organizations need to consider how to organize effectively licensing and reimbursements for personalized medicine (Shane 2007). Therapeutic innovations will have to be introduced without sacrificing patient safety; and so far few adequate policy solutions have been proposed.

- Drug development and approval aiming to improve quality of life need different approaches in terms of assessing cost–effectiveness and cost-benefit. Previous parameters, such as narrow clinical outcomes, are insufficient. Evaluating efficacy, effectiveness or cost–effectiveness must be supplemented, within rigorously conducted trials, by patient-related parameters, such as satisfaction and quality of life. The responsible policy-makers must adapt their licensing and reimbursement schemes accordingly.

- The required evaluation should not block authorization and implementation of new pharmaceuticals and medical devices, but be conducted as quickly as possible.

7.2 Financial incentives

When discussing quality of care, health professionals tend to stress the importance of professional ethos, motivation, adequate staffing levels, and education and training. Research indicates that these dimensions are limited in their capacity to change behaviour (Busse and Mays 2008). Instruments allowing more rapid change are needed, and one of the tools available is financial incentives.

Using financial incentives effectively often means eliminating incentives that make chronic care or disease management less effective, but, however motivated stakeholders may be to improve chronic care, few will operate against their economic interest (Leatherman, Berwick and Iles 2003).

Financial flows influence most of the relationships in a health system, that is, they act as incentives – with intended or unintended effects. This section attempts to define the financial flows/incentives between patients, providers, financial poolers and payers/purchasers. It also examines the intentions and (theoretical) justifications behind these flows, and the results thus far.

Financial incentives can be used to target certain processes or outcome-related goals, but this can be challenging. The treatment needs of patients are complex, and effective management involves a range of people across different sectors. The aim of this section is to give policy-makers the insights they need to think critically about designing financial incentives. First, we identify different financial mechanisms in the health system. Second, we present different types of financial incentives and review the evidence on their impact. Third, we offer some policy recommendations.

Financial mechanisms in health systems

Given the complexity of most health systems, we need a model that will analyse the financial mechanisms as well as show policy-makers how to create a design that will improve care for those with chronic diseases. Busse and Mays (2008) recently developed the **extended triangular model**. It distinguishes between population/payers, providers and financial intermediaries. The latter are subdivided into **financial poolers** and **payers/purchasers** (Fig. 7.1).

This analytical framework allows us to group financial mechanisms and incentives in the following way:

- **Relationship A**: patient —> provider: cost sharing, co-payments

- **Relationship B**: population —> financial pooler: resource generation through taxes, contributions or premiums

- **Relationship C**: financial pooler —> payer/purchaser: (re-)allocations to payer/purchaser

- **Relationship D**: payer/purchaser —> provider: provider remuneration

Fig. 7.1 *Financial relations between stakeholders in health care*

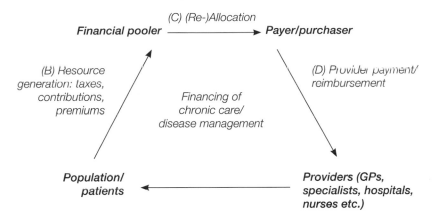

(C) (Re-)Allocation

Financial pooler ⟶ *Payer/purchaser*

(B) Resource generation: taxes, contributions, premiums

Financing of chronic care/ disease management

(D) Provider payment/ reimbursement

Population/ patients

Providers (GPs, specialists, hospitals, nurses etc.)

(A) Cost sharing and direct payments

Source: Busse and Mays 2008.

Currently the main debate is how to remunerate providers (Relationship D). This is central to the discussion in this section. But the other three relationships will also be discussed.

Provider remuneration in chronic care

There are currently three different approaches to paying health professionals from pooled resources, described here.

1. **Capitation** gives the health professional a fixed sum to care for patients over a period of time, irrespective of the services provided. Financial poolers and payers/providers find it easy to budget under this type of payment, but the financial incentives for the health professional can create cause for concern. The danger is that they will offer as little a service as possible to each patient because they are bearing the cost. Services may become underused. Capitation may have worse outcomes for chronic care. Unless there are risk adjustments, providers will not be interested in treating these patients because the cost to them will be more than a capitation sum based on average patients (Busse and Mays 2008).

2. **Fee for service** involves paying for each unit of service provided. It is generally assumed that more services will be provided where margins are high in order to maximize income. This may lead to some services being overused. The effect on chronic care is two-fold. On the one hand, overprovision may be counterproductive. On the other hand, given sensible payments, there are no

incentives for underuse. The fee-for-service approach can also be applied to pay institutions rather than individuals and, in this case, the incentive structure works in the same way.

3. **The salary approach** splits the cost of health care into one part human resource and one part covering other costs. The health professional is compensated by a fixed amount, irrespective of productivity. There is no specific incentive for underuse or overuse of services. At the same time there is no specific incentive to provide good care for chronic patients with chronic illnesses (Busse and Mays 2008).

At the institutional level, approaches include **per diem** payments and **case fees.** Per diem payments (a standard amount per patient per day) have a negative effect on chronic disease. Institutions tend to avoid chronic patients because of their high cost, or keep them in hospital longer than necessary in order to make up the costs through higher overall reimbursement.

Case fees were used originally to pay fixed amounts for each patient with a certain diagnosis. Early systems in the United States assumed that all patients in each diagnosis-related group (DRG) generated similar costs, thus sharing financial risk with providers. This led to seriously ill patients with chronic or multiple diseases being avoided, and also resulted in premature discharge. Approaches in France, Germany and the Netherlands (Busse, Zentner and Schlette 2006) defined outliers with higher payments and based their classifications on hospital procedures. This turned European DRGs into a hybrid with the fee-for-service approach. This reduces adverse selection, but risks overprovision. Institutional budgets have similar incentives for professional salaries. The effect on chronic care will depend on specific arrangements in each context.

Getting financial incentives for providers in line: new initiatives

Beyond these "traditional" approaches, a new set of tools for paying providers has been developed in Europe. Table 7.2 summarizes the main methods by means of which payers can encourage appropriate chronic disease care. Financial incentives can apply to structure, processes and outcomes.

Financial incentives aimed at improving chronic care tend to focus on the structure, processes and outcomes of care (Busse and Mays 2008), but there are regional differences. Most financial incentives in European countries relate to the structure or process of care. Only the United Kingdom NHS contract for GPs specifically includes incentive payments focused on the delivery of particular outcomes (Smith and York 2004; Roland 2004). Generally, the focus has been shifting from approaches which simply take into account the presence (or potential presence) of patients with chronic disease towards funding incentives designed to encourage providers to make specific structural and process responses (Glasgow et al. 2008; Bodenheimer, Wagner and Grumbach 2002a, 2002b).

Table 7.2 *Incentives used to improve chronic care in European countries*

Financial incentives targeting the *individual*	Financial incentives targeting *structures* of care	Financial incentives targeting *processes* of care	Financial incentives targeting *outcomes* of care
• Piloting of "year of care" payment for the complete package of chronic disease management required by individuals with chronic conditions (e.g. based on validated "care pathways" for diabetes) (Denmark, United Kingdom)	• Per-patient bonus for physicians for acting as gatekeepers for chronic patients and for setting care protocols (France) • Bonus for DMP recruitment and documentation (Germany) • 1% of overall health budget available for integrated care (Germany)	• Points for reaching process targets (United Kingdom: GP contract) • Points for reaching outcome targets (United Kingdom: GP contract)	• Points for reaching structural targets (United Kingdom: GP contract)
	• Additional services (e.g. patient self-management education) only reimbursable if physicians and patients participate in DMP (Germany)		

Source: Based on Busse and Mays 2008.

There are only a few good studies of the impact of different payments on quality and/or efficiency of care for chronic disease. Many generate their conclusions individual cases rather than from comparative studies. It is difficult to draw firm conclusions on effectiveness or cost–effectiveness.

Studies of financial incentives for providers in Europe have tended to suggest that clear conclusions are impossible because of a lack of evidence. One United States study (Petersen et al. 2006) generated some preliminary conclusions and these might be used to inform the European debate. Their conclusions are discussed here.

• Designs setting out a few narrow goals may lead to excessive focus on the incentivized tasks or areas of quality, generating "gaming" or better reporting without any true improvements in care quality. These problems are well documented in other sectors (Baron and Kreps 1999).

• The impact of financial incentives is not the same for different groups of providers. Those with high, average or poor performance will each react differently.

- Mixed approaches combining different payment schemes (such as fee for service and case fees) may reduce the negative effects of either approach applied alone.

- The size of the incentives clearly matters. Studies in other sectors suggest that a significant percentage of income has to be variable before providers can be expected to change their behaviour. Overly large incentives, on the other hand, may lead to providers focusing too much on incentivized goals.

- Motivational theory suggests that financial incentives will be less effective for groups of providers than they will be for individuals (Baron and Kreps 1999). This is because the individual's effort is only partly reflected in group benefits, with some colleagues earning the same for less work carried out. As a result, individuals are less motivated to improve quality. On the other hand, at the provider-group level, risk-adjustment can take place, which is not possible for individuals.

- Small to medium-sized multidisciplinary teams tend to provide positive outcomes (Bodenheimer, Wagner and Grumbach 2002a, 2002b), suggesting that this could be an appropriate way of providing financial incentives to providers, especially when combined with rigorous performance monitoring and benchmarking (Kerr and Fleming 2007).

Clearly, one cannot deduce that these conclusions apply in the European context, but they offer a good starting point for future investigation.

Some evidence has been generated about the Quality and Outcomes Framework (QOF) in the United Kingdom, which set up "pay for performance" for GPs, using outcomes and quality variables and making about 25% of practice income dependent on quality rewards. The programme is still controversial, but in general it has had a positive effect on quality of care, and particularly chronic care (Campbell, Reeves and Kontopantelis 2007). Most researchers conclude that improvements are likely to be the result of better organization of general practices. In particular, it seems that patients benefit from more systematic care (Wang et al. 2006).

Financial incentives for payers/purchasers

Few policy approaches use financial incentives to target payers and/or purchasers. One exception is the 2002 health reform in Germany, which changed the method of allocating individual sickness funds. Before the reform, it was unattractive to insure patients with chronic diseases or to set up DMPs for people with chronic illnesses. After the reform, sickness funds received extra funding when enrolling patients in DMPs. This led to a rapid growth of such programmes. No systematic reviews on the impact of these programmes on health outcomes or the use of resources have yet been published. Some critics have already attacked the formula on the grounds that putting people into DMPs does not necessarily mean that they get better care (see section 5.3).

Another health reform in Germany, implemented in January 2009, provides extra financial incentives for payers and insurers by taking individual morbidity criteria into account (individually risk-rated capitations) (Schang 2009). A similar scheme – although encompassing fewer diseases – was implemented in the Netherlands (Van Ginneken, Busse and Gericke 2008).

Financial incentives for patients

There are relatively few financial incentives for patients to take part in chronic DMPs. France and Germany are exceptions because they apply (modest) cost-sharing mechanisms. Cost sharing may be reduced or waived in Germany when patients enrol in a programme. This incentive was mainly used to attract people to take part in DMPs. Patients taking part also have access to extra services. Patients in France become exempt from co-payments for chronic disease care if they present their previously agreed care protocol at every physician visit. Neither scheme has yet been systematically analysed.

Financial incentives for promoting better chronic disease management are rarely used to affect the relationship between financial poolers and the population (relationship B in Fig. 7.1). One such incentive would be to lower premiums or contribution rates for those with chronic diseases who take part in a DMP. There are no such schemes in Europe.

Policy recommendations

This section demonstrates that early findings suggest that financial incentives can be used to promote better quality care when properly applied and when certain prerequisites are fulfilled. The section makes recommendations for policy-makers considering new financial incentives. It builds on the findings discussed and incorporates relevant findings from other sections. It separates structural and operational recommendations.

Structural policy recommendations

• Most European countries have set up programmes to promote chronic disease management, but these programmes rarely give financial compensation to integrated approaches targeting several chronic diseases. Research shows that chronic illnesses and chronic conditions are increasingly interrelated (Busse and Mays 2008). Policy-makers as well as decision-makers within public and private institutions should therefore consider integrating or linking chronic care programmes.

• Continuity of care is a key prerequisite for payer or provider investment in chronic DMPs. Any net returns from investments in infrastructure tend to become available five years later (Suhrcke, Fahey and McKee 2008); and benefits from avoiding severe complications are evident after 5–10 years (Eastman et al. 1997). Health systems that have traditionally focused on "patient choice", and include little enrolment with particular providers and/or fee-for-service payments – all of which have led to relatively poor continuity of care – face the greatest difficulties in aligning financial incentives to promote better management. With this in mind, policy-makers should consider strengthening or introducing financial incentives at all levels that will encourage "continuity of care".

• In most European countries, different professional groups are paid according to separate schemes. However, effective care often depends on the cooperation of multidisciplinary teams. Different incentives for different members of the same team may frustrate common efforts, where economic interests motivate different treatments. Policy-makers should align compensation schemes across different sectors for health professionals working together in the chronic care sector.

Operational policy recommendations

• Financial incentives encouraging a few narrow goals can lead to excessive focus on these goals, together with "gaming" or better reporting without any improvements in quality. Policy-makers as well as health care managers should set out quality indicators that reflect different aspects of quality (structure, process and, where possible, outcome).

• Since the impact of financial incentives is likely to differ across different groups of providers, policy-makers should decide which they want to incentivize and then design the incentives accordingly.

• Policy-makers should consider mixed payment approaches, since this can mitigate negative effects of individual approaches.

• Theory and empirical evidence suggest that a substantial amount of income has to be variable before providers can be expected to change their behaviour. Incentives should not therefore be too large, given the sensitivity of quality in health care and lack of clarity about the impact of different payment schemes. Where possible, pilot studies should be conducted before programmes are rolled out.

- Financial incentives for individuals may undermine cooperation, while financial incentives for organizations may have little impact on the motivation of individuals. Using small-to-medium multidisciplinary teams seems to yield positive outcomes (Bodenheimer, Wagner and Grumbach 2002a, 2002b), so policy-makers should consider targeting these groups when introducing financial incentives.

7.3 Improving coordination

Research suggests that one of the major obstacles to better care for those with chronic disease is the lack of coordination in health care systems. Structured approaches, such as DMPs and integrated multi-disease care models tend to fall between different layers of increasingly differentiated health systems (Busse 2004; Epping-Jordan et al. 2004; Velasco-Garrido, Busse and Hisashige 2003; Pelikan and Nowak 1998). This section examines different ways of coordinating services, along with the structural, organizational and operational barriers. Finally, it makes recommendations so that policy-makers can define strategies for better coordination.

Dimensions of coordination in chronic care

Clearly, involving more providers requires better coordination. Chronic care often involves multi-provider settings, and since patients with chronic conditions often have several diseases, coordination is particularly appropriate. Research confirms that patients' perception of the quality of care is largely determined by how successful this coordination is. The following dimensions are important:

- **getting in** – getting access to appropriate care;
- **fitting in** – adapting the care to their requirements;
- **knowing what is going on** – receiving information;
- **continuity** – of staff and also coordination and communication among professionals; and
- difficulties in making **progress** through the system, mainly due to failures in the other four areas (Preston et al. 1999).

Boon and colleagues (2004) identified seven types of provision with varying degrees of coordination (Fig. 7.2). At one end of the continuum is **strict solo provision**. At the other end is **full integration of disciplines** for curative, rehabilitative and preventive services. Second on the non-coordination side of the continuum is **parallel practice**, whereby practitioners work independently and carry out services independently. **Consultative practice** is where information on patients is shared informally, case by case. In **coordinated practice** the exchange of data on patients is related to particular diseases, and therapies are administered through a formal structure. Often a case coordinator will supervise the exchange of patient records. An advanced model of the former is the **multidisciplinary team**, which is more formalized, has more team members, and often clear team structures with sub-teams and team leaders. An **interdisciplinary team** is one in which group decisions are made, shared policies developed, and regular face-to-face meetings held. Finally, **integrative practice** is based on a shared vision and provides a "seamless continuum of decision-making and patient-centred care and support".

Fig. 7.2 *Types of care provision with varying degrees of coordination*

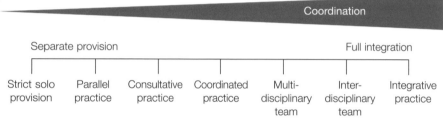

Source: Based on Boon et al. 2004.

Barriers to coordination

The problems of coordinating health care systems have been the subject of wide-ranging discussions for decades (Grundmeyer 1996). We concentrate on structural as well as organizational and operational problems.

Structural problems of coordination

Structural problems are often rooted in different ways of working across different sectors (primary or secondary; public or private). Providers are faced with incentives to compete rather than to cooperate. Individuals or professional groups are compensated for separate activities rather than for cooperation. There is rivalry over resources and power struggles between professional groups, as well as overlapping responsibilities and unclear accountability between divisions and providers. Box 7.1 summarizes common structural barriers in Europe.

These problems exist to varying degrees in most European health systems, but different problems arise in countries where general practice has a central gatekeeping position. Gatekeeping is designed to promote integration and coordination of care provision (Calnan, Hutten and Tiljak 2006). The various coordination problems are summarized in the following subsections.

Box 7.1 *Structural barriers to coordination*

- Competing operation cultures and management approaches in different sectors (social care versus health care; primary sector versus secondary sector; home practice versus general practice)
- Different ownership structures (lack of universal standard for the interfaces between the public and the private sectors)
- Separate and competing providers with no incentives to cooperate
- Rivalries between professional groups
- Lack of clarity about competencies and accountability (national versus regional actors for policy initiatives; general practice versus specialists for the process of care)

Source: Based on Nolte and McKee 2008.

Structural problems of coordination in gatekeeping countries

In gatekeeping countries, general practice guides patients through the health care system. Those entitled to regular care are registered with a general practice and the GP has access to their records. General practice is usually the first point of access, irrespective of medical problem or need. Other providers, such as specialists, are only accessible after consultation with or referral by the GP. Drugs tend to be provided by prescription only. In this context general practice has two main roles: (1) controlling the use of specialist services, which is meant to reduce or contain health care costs; and (2) acting as a coordinator, providing navigation and continuity of care, as well as encouraging the system to be more responsive (Calnan, Hutten and Tiljak 2006). This latter function should benefit patients with chronic disease, because different professionals are involved at different stages and continuity of care is essential.

Nevertheless, the record relating to gatekeeping approaches in providing better coordination is mixed. Some evaluations have found that gatekeeping approaches are successful (Gervas, Perez-Fernandez and Starfield 1994; Gross, Tabenkin and Brammli-Greenberg 2000; Engström, Foldevi and Borgquist 2001; Starfield, Shi and Macinko 2005), while others suggest that there is no conclusive evidence that gatekeeping contains health care costs or enhances the quality of care (Martin et al. 1989; Meyer et al. 1996). There are several reasons for the contradictions: implementation and operational problems (which will be discussed in more detail here), and context-specific structural problems. For example, in many countries the role of GPs is unclear once the patient has passed through the gate into the rest of the system (Calnan, Hutten and Tiljak 2006). Also, conflicts rooted in the traditional hierarchy of the medical professions may undermine the success of gatekeeping models. General practice is often at the lower end of the doctors' hierarchy, even though the gatekeeping model places them in a central position. The new "governance" model challenges the well-established hierarchy, and may lead to conflicts regarding legitimacy, power and resources. Depending on their intensity, these conflicts may lead to less rather than more coordination among various professionals.

Structural problems of coordination in non-gatekeeping countries

Coordination problems are different in countries with no gatekeepers. Patients can visit a GP or specialist without a referral. If they prescribe tests or elements of care, patients usually have the right to choose who should carry this out. It is not necessary to be registered with one general practice. Patients have a greater choice of providers, but no individual health professional is responsible for the full process. Navigation through the system and through different stages of care is not part of the system, so patients have to organize their own pathway. This can result in serious problems, particularly regarding continuity of care. France, for example, did not introduce gatekeeping to promote navigation through the health system until 2005. Evaluations indicated that this was not good for chronic care. Treatment for diabetes, for example, was fragmented (Bras, Duhamel and Grass 2006) and, as a result, national guidelines were only rarely respected (Calnan, Hutten and Tiljak 2006).

Organizational and operational problems of coordination

In addition to structural problems, the following organizational and operational aspects impede effective coordination.

Funding and finance

Some European countries have invested considerably to improve chronic care, but those measures intended to increase cooperation are often discontinued after early success. Governments seem to expect that measures to improve coordination will "self-fund" from savings (Leutz 1999). However, evaluations show that these expectations are unrealistic, and threaten the success of efforts to improve coordination. In many cases, "self-funding" expectations are seen as a threat by those within the organization, particularly if ambitious savings are expected. They may fear that they will have to make the "efficiency gains" by cutting resources. Given strong incentives to protect these resources, willingness to cooperate has been found to be low (Leutz 1999).

Research also indicates that coordination initiatives seldom generate short-term savings. In addition, improving coordination does not compensate for a lack of resources (Freeman, Woloshynowych and Baker 2007), and so is not an easy way to solve funding problems.

Human resources and pay

Integrated approaches (such as DMPs or gatekeeping models) that bridge traditional professional boundaries need well-defined roles and competences (Nolte and McKee 2008). In many countries, legal boundaries have to be redrawn before competences can shift between professional groups (Durand-Zaleski and Obrecht 2008). Reimbursement schemes have to be adapted in order to compensate participation in new schemes, such as multidisciplinary teams to treat chronic diseases (Glasgow et al. 2008). The evidence clearly shows that professional groups will be less involved in integrated care models unless they have pay incentives (Steuten et al. 2002; Schiøtz, Frølich and Krasnik 2008).

In addition, performance-related pay schemes may set incentives which undermine cooperation (Hofmarcher, Oxley and Rusticelli 2007). Specialist doctors are particularly worried about shifting competences to other professional groups, such as nurses or GPs, and this can undermine coordination of chronic care (Rosemann, Joest and Koerner 2006). The lack of training for staff undertaking new roles is a serious problem. Doctors in most countries are rarely trained to "navigate" patients through the health system. Nurses having to perform new and demanding tasks are often inadequately prepared and supported.

Strategies for better coordination

Policy-makers increasingly recognize the importance of coordination for the quality of care (Boerma 2006), patients' care experience (Alazri et al. 2006; Schoen, Osborn and Doty 2007; Turner, Tarrant and Windridge 2007) and cost-containment. Accordingly, governments in most European countries have developed appropriate strategies.

Many of these strategies have been applied to the structural, organizational and operational problems of coordination. Some countries, such as Denmark and England, have developed national strategies for chronic care, integrating health promotion, prevention and management under a common framework. Other countries, where professionals are more fragmented, have developed strategies focusing on specific aspects of chronic care and chronic disease (France, Germany, the Netherlands and Sweden) (Nolte and McKee 2008).

Table 7.3 summarizes recent policy initiatives in selected European countries. It distinguishes between those with a common framework and thus a **national strategy**, and those using **parallel strategies**.

Table 7.3 *Recent policy initiatives to improve coordination and quality of chronic care*

Country	Policy initiatives	Goals/mechanisms
Denmark	**National strategy**	
	• Development of a national vision of chronic disease control: Healthy throughout life (2002) • National targets to increase life expectancy • Reallocation of responsibilities between regions and municipalities • Municipal health centres for the elderly and patients with chronic disease (limited to the provision of non-physician services)	• Facilitate easier access to chronic care via municipal centres • Increase transparency and accountability via defined targets
France	**Parallel strategies**	
	• Introduction of "health networks" • Target-setting for health and risk indicators • Universal and mandatory registration with GP • Financial incentives (reduction of co-payments) for the use of evidence-based guidelines in provision of long-term conditions	• Improve exchange of experience between providers via networks • Increase transparency and accountability via defined targets • Increase the use of evidence-based guidelines in chronic care via financial incentives • Improve navigation through the system via universal gatekeeping by general practice
Germany	**Parallel strategies**	
	• Attractive compensation for DMPs (2002 and 2004)	• Establish integrated and structured care models via attractive financial compensation for the establishment of DMPs
Netherlands	**Parallel strategies**	
	• Establishment of transmural care (focusing on the interface between acute hospital care and alternative setting) • Development of DMPs	• Improving the interface between acute hospital care and ambulatory care via new initiatives/cooperation between existing actors in transmural care • Development of integrated care models via financial for the establishment of DMPs
Sweden[a]	**Parallel strategies**	
	• Strong emphasis on primary care centres for chronic care guided by regional and local guidelines • Nurse-led chronic care • Development of chains of care • Development of "local health care" initiatives	• Improve navigation, accessibility and continuity of care via chronic care in primary care centres and nurse-led chronic care • Improve quality of chronic care via the development of common guidelines for chronic care across professional and provider boundaries ("chains of care") • Increase continuity of care and accessibility for elderly and patients with chronic disease via locally coordinated health care strategies

Table 7.3 *cont.*

United Kingdom	*National strategy*	
	• Development of a national vision for chronic care: Choosing Health (2004) • Implementation of case management • Risk stratification • Multidisciplinary care teams • New payment system for primary care • Establishment of "NHS walk-in centres" and "NHS Direct"	• Improve navigation through the system via case management • Define adequate policies for patients via stratification and clustering • Develop integrated chronic care via multidisciplinary teams • Establish the provision of high-quality care for selected chronic conditions in primary practice via a new compensation scheme • Increase access to chronic care for specific patient groups via multiple points of entry

Sources: Authors' own compilation based on Nolte and McKee 2008 and on Calnan, Hutten and Tiljak 2006.
[a] Sweden devolves significant responsibility for health care to provinces and other lower levels of government. Therefore policy approaches differ across the country. These are only selected policy initiatives.

Despite these initiatives, problems with coordination and continuity of care persist, irrespective of the health care system and the policy approach (Calnan, Hutten and Tiljak 2006). Given the lack of research, short duration of the initiatives and relationship to country-specific variables, only tentative conclusions can be drawn. One is that, while gatekeeping countries such as the Netherlands and the United Kingdom still have problems of coordination and continuity of care, these problems tend to be worse in health systems with no systematic gatekeeping and where patients are left to navigate through the system on their own.

Furthermore, many governments try to improve the coordination of services in primary, specialist and social care, of community services through joint committees, and of shared care. Evaluations suggest that the success of these approaches is limited and depends on the cooperation of different professionals (Evans 1996).

Finally, increasing points of entry to the system via **walk-in centres** or **call-in centres** comes at a cost. It tends to split primary care and undermine continuity of care (Anderson et al. 2002; Salisbury 2004). For some patients, especially those with chronic and multiple conditions, this may make it harder to improve quality of care (Calnan et al. 1994).

Policy recommendations

There is no agreed best practice for better coordination. Problems persist in all European health systems and the impacts of various policies differ. Formulating policy is difficult, but studies have informed the following recommendations.

Strategic policy recommendations

• Governments and policy-makers across sectors must recognize that they need to act. The complexity and variety of people involved in chronic care means that better coordination will not emerge spontaneously (Nolte and McKee 2008). Decision-makers must make better cooperation a priority in order to overcome deeply rooted vested interests and professional scepticism. Better coordination will only become a realistic goal if it is adequately managed and politically supported.

• Policy-makers must decide early whether change can be implemented in the existing system, or whether fundamental reform is needed. This applies particularly where there are central structural barriers to cooperation (Glasgow et al. 2008; Nolte and McKee 2008; Plochg and Klazinga 2002).

• All European health systems face increasing demands on health outcomes, medical progress and finances. Policy-makers should take into account the consequences of restructuring when designing policies specifically targeting coordination (Nolte and McKee 2008).

Structural policy recommendations

• Governments should decide what mix of **centrally controlled parameters** and **local autonomy**, or **top-down** and **bottom-up** management they wish to implement in order to improve coordination (Åhgren and Axelsson 2007). Policy-makers must take into account the likelihood of bringing about change. They should also consider whether their approach will integrate with established mechanisms of accountability and responsiveness. In Germany, strict national guidelines for DMPs have been praised for ensuring common standards, but they have also been criticized for making it difficult to respond to local requirements and conditions (Siering 2008). In England, a perceived lack of regulation has been blamed as the main cause of a highly differentiated and fragmented set of programmes.

• Similarly, policy-makers should choose between **parallel policy initiatives** or one **integrated national strategy**.

• Key actors should decide which patient group they wish to target. The debate regarding whether to increase access through multiple entry points or to strengthen continuity of care and improve navigation with gatekeeping shows that policies to improve chronic care often involve trade-offs for different groups of patients. Policy-makers should define the target (patient) population of their strategies in order to minimize unintended consequences and side-effects.

- Separate and shared responsibilities within and between providers should be clearly defined in order to prevent duplication or omissions (Calnan, Hutten and Tiljak 2006).

Organizational and operational policy recommendations

- In all sectors, policy-makers should provide enough funding to cover start-up costs and sustained operations. Expectations of self-funding tend to be unrealistic and often engender rivalry over resources (Leutz 1999).

- Policy-makers should set up remuneration schemes that will allow cooperation across primary and secondary sectors, professional groups and competing providers.

- Policy-makers should enable health professionals to fulfil their new responsibilities. This involves setting up an appropriate legal framework, providing training, and helping to build trust between professional groups that are not used to working together.

7.4 Information and communication technology

There is growing international agreement that introducing modern ICT may lead to more effective use of resources, an improvement in quality of care, and greater attention paid to the needs and wishes of patients (Busse, Zentner and Schlette 2006). In particular, DMPs and integrated care models need strong and effective systems for exchanging information and collecting data if they want to achieve constant quality control (Hofmarcher, Oxley and Rusticelli 2007; Leutz 1999).

The European Union (EU) has therefore proposed various information technology initiatives – for example, within the framework of the eEurope action plan (now called i2010) – and many governments have been motivated to intensify their efforts (European Commission 2009). For the health sector, the EU presented the eHealth action plan, which encourages Member States to develop their e-health strategies. It also seeks to set up agreed international standards for exchanging health data (European Commission 2004). This section will give policy-makers an overview of the effectiveness of different decision-support systems. It will also highlight how various countries are reforming their e-health platforms and electronic health records.

Clinical decision support systems

Clinical decision-making is supported by a wide range of interventions. These rely increasingly on electronic systems for their delivery. The main goals are to increase the quality of care by standardizing the delivery of care in accordance with evidence-based practice, while at the same time containing costs (Glasgow et al. 2008). Clinical care processes are more likely to become standardized when evidence-based practice guidelines or protocols and clinical pathways are being used. They are intended to reduce variation in health care and thereby increase quality of outcomes and reduce medical error. Coiera (2003) points out that these electronic systems range from presenting information (treatment requirements for specific conditions or diagnosis) to undertaking complex functions, as is the case with **expert systems** and **machine learning systems**. Evidence suggests that formal decision-support systems are beneficial, and they have been studied for conditions such as hypertension, diabetes, depression, heart failure, asthma, COPD, osteoarthritis and end-stage renal failure.

Table 7.4 summarizes the evidence of effectiveness of decision support in clinical practice.

The evidence so far indicates that progress has been made in some disease areas. Nevertheless, many challenges remain if we are to make full use of the potential of decision supports (Glasgow et al. 2008).

E-health platforms and electronic health records

Many governments support holistic information and communications systems such as e-health platforms and electronic health records or cards. The aim is to improve data exchange between key people such as doctors, patients, hospital workers, pharmacists, care workers, health insurers and public administrators. E-health platforms are intended to improve access, increase patient participation, improve efficiency of delivery and improve coordination. Often the platforms incorporate guidelines for professionals, information and education programmes for patients, and eligibility criteria detailing benefits.

Examples of such platforms include the Canadian Health Infoway, MedCom in Denmark, NHS Connecting for Health in Britain, Health Connect Australia and an Internet portal in France for chronic conditions (Glasgow et al. 2008). Cross-sectoral electronic health records are used for the long-term collection and documentation of relevant patients. They contain personal data and a wealth of medical information, such as the medical history of the patient, laboratory results, physicians' letters, records of operations and digital data from investigations (Busse, Zentner and Schlette 2006). Only a small amount of evidence is available, but some studies have found positive effects on the care process, while others have found no effect on subjective or objective outcomes (O'Connor, Lauren Crain and Rush 2005; Tierney, Overhage and Murray 2005).

Table 7.4 *Evidence of effectiveness: clinical decision support system (CDSS)*

Study with (abbreviated) title and source	Study design	Condition/ treatment	Target	Type of intervention	Patient objective outcomes	Patient subjective outcomes	Quality of care	Reduced health care costs/use of services
Effects of CDSS systems (Garg, Adhikari and McDonald 2005)	Systematic review	n/a	Practitioner	CDSS		+		
Decision aids for people facing health treatment or screening decisions[a] (O'Connor, Stacey and Entwistle 2003)	Systematic review	n/a	Patients	Computer and web-based decision aids	+		-	
Effect of computerized evidence-based guidelines on management of asthma and angina in adults (Eccles, McColl and Steen 2002)	RCT	Asthma, angina	GP	Computerized guidelines	-	-	-	-
Effect of computer-aided management on the quality of treatment in anticoagulated patients (Manotti, Moia and Palareti 2001)	RCT	Oral anticoagulant treatment	Anticoagulant clinic physicians	Computer-aided dosing	+		+	+
A randomized trial using CDSS to improve treatment of major depression in primary care (Rollman, Hanusa and Lowe 2002)	RCT	Major depression	GP	CDSS with diagnostic and feedback on treatment	-		-	
Lessons from a RCT designed to evaluate CDSS software to improve the management of asthma (McCowan, Neville and Ricketts 2001)	RCT	Asthma	GP	CDSS	~			~
Failure of computerized treatment suggestions to improve health outcomes of outpatients with uncomplicated hypertension (Murray, Harris and Overhage 2004)	RCT	Hypertension	Physicians, pharmacists	Evidence-based treatment suggestions using eHR	-	-	-	

Table 7.4 cont.

Can computer-generated evidence care suggestions enhance evidence-based management of asthma and COPD? (Tierney, Overhagy and Murray 2005)	RCT	Asthma, COPD	GP	Computer-based evidence care suggestions	–	–	–
RCT of an informatics-based intervention to increase statin prescription for secondary prevention of coronary disease (Lester et al. 2006)	RCT	Ischaemic heart disease	GP	CDSS	+	+	
Cost-effectiveness of an intervention based on the GINA recommendations using a CDSS system (Plaza, Cobos and Ignacio-Garcia 2005)	RCT	Asthma	Specialist and GP	CDSS	+	+	

Source: Glasgow et al. 2008.

Notes: "+": Intervention improves the outcome; "?": Intervention does not show any effect on the outcome; "–": Intervention has a negative effect on the outcome; * The majority of studies included in this review concerned cancer screening and treatment; 25% of the decision aids reviewed were not computer/web-based – however, the review provides important evidence on the use of decision aids for patients and was therefore included here. n/a: not applicable; RCT: Randomized controlled trial; GINA: Global Initiative for Asthma; eHR: electronic health records.

In addition, the European Commission places great hope on telemedicine applications such as telemonitoring and teleradiology "for the benefit of patients, healthcare systems and society", though it admits that "there is limited evidence of the effectiveness and cost–effectiveness of telemedicine services on a large scale" (European Commission 2008). The Communication issued in 2008 aims at strengthening "awareness, confidence and acceptance by health authorities, professionals and patients".

Policy recommendations

- Agreeing on technical standards is essential because one of the key challenges is to achieve functional interoperability within health systems. Policy-makers at government level and within regulating bodies in the different health systems should bring those involved together and ensure that they agree on goals and standards for information technology.

- More important is how the vast amounts of data generated by medical treatments can be merged into meaningful information. Modern information technology can store vast amounts of data, but health professionals usually need carefully selected pieces of information combined in a specific way. Since time is critical, both in terms of costs and medical treatment, intelligent ways of condensing, aggregating and interpreting information must be found. ICT providers often ignore this, but high-level policy-makers should insist that systems are developed in order to meet the needs of health professionals.

- The use of information technology should be more broadly evaluated. Pilot projects in Austria, Canada, France, Germany, Italy, Japan, Switzerland and the United States have found relatively high costs, budget overruns and many unforeseen difficulties (Hendy et al. 2005; Tuffs 2004; Tuffs 2006; Burton, Anderson and Kues 2004; Scott et al. 2005). There is a clear need to assess the benefits of information technology and long-term cost–benefit analyses should be undertaken.

- Policy-makers and health care professionals at all levels should ensure that patients accept the new electronic systems. Data protection is a key part of new designs, but patients often demand full access to their own data. Where necessary, laws must be passed to ensure strict standards on data protection, and to affirm patients' rights to access their records.

7.5 Evaluation culture

We have shown that many strategies and interventions have not yet been properly evaluated and neither their effectiveness nor their cost–effectiveness have been established. Policy-makers for chronic care lack high-quality information based on scientifically valid methods to support their decisions. This section outlines how technologies (medical devices and pharmaceuticals) and strategies are evaluated in different countries, describes what methodology should be used and outlines which steps could be taken to improve evaluations.

Evaluation is described here as the comparative appraisal of technologies and strategies used to manage chronic disease – pharmaceuticals, programmes, projects, services or organizations – using methodically aggregated and analysed data (Øvretveit 1998). The evaluation can relate to the structure, process and results of an intervention. Evidence-based assessment and quality development must be transparent and must provide the conditions necessary for rational health planning and control (Busse, Zentner and Schlette 2006). Unlike basic research, evaluation addresses the specific questions of decision-makers on efficacy, cost–effectiveness and equity.

Evaluation of medical procedures and devices

Evaluating chronic disease management requires careful preparation and should be built into a programme from the start. However, few countries have adopted the idea that evaluation should be an integral part of public health programmes. Exceptions include the Netherlands, Canada, Australia and the United Kingdom (Suhrcke, Fahey and McKee 2008). Since the 1990s the global trend has been more towards evidence-based policy. Many countries are trying to evaluate medical technologies and procedures, for instance, including those for chronic diseases. This is usually carried out by health technology assessment (HTA) institutions. Most European HTA agencies are independent of government but are publicly funded, with the mandate of supporting policy-making and decision-making. An increasing number of European countries can draw on their experiences evaluating health technologies and supporting policy decisions (Velasco-Garrido et al. 2008).

Evaluation of pharmaceuticals

People with multiple diseases are becoming much more complex to manage as new, more powerful, but also potentially more dangerous drugs become available (Nolte and McKee 2008). Until recently, there was only limited evidence for the pharmacological management of chronic disease. That was particularly the case for new drugs that had proven their safety and efficacy in randomized controlled trials (RCTs – often against a placebo as a control) and were licensed to be marketed. But it was unclear whether they offered any additional benefits – especially in real-life conditions – over existing pharmaceuticals. Were they really innovative, or simply patented "me too" products with no (or very limited) added value?

Many countries have therefore introduced a post-licensing evaluation before making decisions on price, eligibility for reimbursement and recommendations (within clinical guidelines) for use (Zentner, Velasco-Garrido and Busse 2005). The number of groups assessing evidence on the added value of a drug has grown continuously since the late 1990s. Examples of such bodies are the Swiss Federal Office of Public Health and Confederate Pharmaceutical Commission, the Swedish Pharmaceutical Benefits Board Committee and the National Institute for Health and Clinical Excellence in the United Kingdom (Zentner, Velasco-Garrido and Busse 2005).

Negative reviews from these bodies cause the pharmaceutical industry to criticize the lengthy evaluation procedures and the quality of the evidence-based evaluations. Reimbursement decisions have been contested successfully in litigation, for example in France (Naudin and Sermet 2003; Couffinhal 2003). The example of Australia (Van Gool 2005) shows how drug evaluation and regulation increasingly come into conflict with a global market. The free trade agreement with the United States obliges Australia to allow an independent assessor to review rejections by its Pharmaceutical Benefits Advisory Committee. One of the challenges facing policy-makers is to develop internationally accepted standards and methods of evidence-based evaluation, and to increase the transparency of the procedures and of policy decisions (Busse, Zentner and Schlette 2006).

Methods of evaluation

Chronic disease management tries to strike the right balance between scarce resources on the one hand and high-quality health care on the other. If models are to be acceptable, their impact needs to be proven. DMPs, for example, should comply with the standards set out for evidence-based medicine. These standards should also apply to evaluation. Prospective, randomized, controlled evaluation is seen as the best method of generating empirical evidence on health service provision. From a statistical point of view, observational studies are weaker when evaluating the effectiveness of CCMs, even though the observation of a cohort can be larger than an RCT sample size. However, RCTs allow different programmes to be compared, in addition to evaluating one intervention (Sawicki et al. 2006; Beyer et al. 2006).

Developing a study design for an RCT in disease management would face methodological problems. These would include defining primary target criteria, guaranteeing a "naturalistic" intensity of intervention and creating a control group that is not significantly affected by spill-over effects (such as the physicians using knowledge they have gained from the programme or implementation becoming mandatory during the evaluation period). Evaluations considering relevant health outcomes also need a long observation time.

These problems can be addressed scientifically (through cluster randomization with physicians having either only DMP patients or none). However, scientists face challenges when conducting adequate evaluations, because decision-makers need rapid answers and might encourage measuring process rather than outcomes.

Evaluation of strategies in chronic disease management

Evaluating strategies in chronic disease management is a part of health services research. It examines how social factors, financial systems, organizational structures and processes, health technologies and personal behaviours affect access to health care, the quality and cost of health care and, ultimately, the health and well-being of citizens (Lohr and Steinwachs 2002; AcademyHealth 2007). Such evaluation does this at a **macro level**, which is the health care system at large (regionally, nationally or internationally) and at a **micro level**, which is the interaction between patients and providers. HTA concentrates on the micro level when evaluating new pharmaceuticals or medical devices (Velasco-Garrido et al. 2008). The **meso level** focuses on health care organizations and the services they provide, as with DMPs.

Several small-scale research projects are studying individual elements of DMPs, such as patient enrolment or documentation. Until now there have been few large-scale, population-based evaluations of chronic care.

One example is the German ELSID study. In 2003 the first DMPs for patients with diabetes mellitus type 2 were introduced in Germany. The *Social Code Book V* made evaluation obligatory and a prerequisite for further accreditation. The regional health funds commissioned independent scientists to evaluate the DMP for type 2 diabetes in primary care in two German states. They designed a 3-armed prospective cluster-randomized comparison of a DMP; a DMP providing extra services, such as quality circles or outreach visits; and routine care without a DMP as a control group. Fig. 7.3 shows the study design (Joos, Rosemann and Heiderhoff 2005).

This is an example of best practice. It allows valid data to be collected and conclusions drawn about the effectiveness of a DMP. This RCT seems promising.

Fig. 7.3 *ELSID – study design*

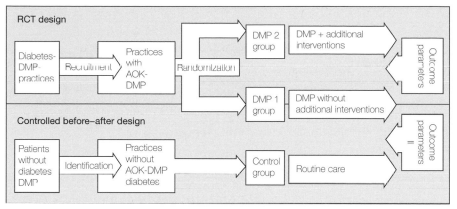

Source: Joos, Rosemann and Heiderhoff 2005.
Note: AOK: General regional health funds.

Policy recommendations

• Policy-makers at government level and within regulatory agencies should understand the relevance and basic methodological requirements of evaluation. They should use this knowledge to ensure that evaluation is an integral part of programmes to improve chronic disease management. Adequate incentives or regulations should be applied to encourage programme designers to take account of the need for evaluation. For example, constant quality control through defined evaluation should be compulsory for large-scale publicly funded programmes.

• Given increasing globalization, policy-makers need to develop internationally agreed standards and methods of evidence-based evaluation. They also need to make their procedures and policy decisions more transparent (Busse, Zentner and Schlette 2006; Sorenson et al. 2008).

• The need for evaluation should not unnecessarily hinder innovation, nor should it be used as an excuse for uncontrolled implementation. Policy-makers must use a step-by-step approach, such as encouraging a small number of providers to use the technology, strategy or organizational component with regard to a small number of patients. Once positive results are available, the number of providers and/or patients may be increased.

• Governments should ensure that data routinely available in different sectors of the health system (for example, for reimbursement) are made available so that independent researchers can carry out in-depth analyses of effectiveness and cost–effectiveness.

Chapter 8
Conclusions

Chronic conditions and diseases are already the leading cause of mortality and morbidity in Europe. Research suggests that conditions such as diabetes and depression will impose an ever larger burden in future.

The economic implications of chronic diseases and conditions are serious. They depress wages, earnings, workforce participation, labour productivity and hours worked – and may also lead to early retirement, high job turnover and disability. Disease-related impairment of household consumption and educational performance affect GDP and economic growth. Spending on chronic care is rising across Europe, and takes up an increasing proportion of public and private budgets.

European policy-makers must undertake serious efforts to tackle chronic disease. In order to inform decision-making, Part I of this book described the available strategies and the evidence on their effectiveness and cost–effectiveness.

In terms of **prevention and early detection**, we have shown that most countries are trying to combat chronic conditions by experimenting with prevention and early detection. These approaches aim to reduce the burden of chronic disease by means of activities that avoid impairment to health, or make it more unlikely. Prevention includes primary, secondary or tertiary approaches which differ in aims and target groups. Research indicates that approaches combining several interventions at once are most effective. Cost–effectiveness analyses indicate that efficient strategies exist to combat chronic disease, but they are rarely more cost-effective than therapeutic interventions. Cost–effectiveness varies considerably according to region and population group. Regional factors for each intervention must be carefully examined, and relevant target groups defined carefully so that policy-makers can do more than just choose between broad implementation or no implementation at all. Prevention interventions are far from developed in most countries. Because of the severe medical, social and economic consequences of chronic diseases, more effort and resources must be invested in prevention and early detection.

Health care has recently seen the emergence of **new providers, new settings and new qualifications**. New professions, such as nurse practitioners, liaison nurses and community nurses have been set up, and the tasks and responsibilities of existing professional groups have been moved and expanded. New settings have been established, such as nurse-led clinics, group practices and medical polyclinics. A key challenge is to enable those working in chronic care to meet their new duties and responsibilities. Some countries have recognized this challenge, but gaps remain. In particular, there is often a shortage of specifically targeted training for those in lower status professions. Empirical evidence on new qualifications and settings is limited, but pilot studies suggest that new qualifications, structures and settings can help to effectively manage chronic diseases. Nurses with wider roles and clinics run by specialist nurses seem to improve chronic care. The cost–effectiveness of such measures has rarely been studied systematically, but some research indicates that use of resources improves. Future research should build on these early results to decide whether investment is justified and where the priorities should lie.

DMPs have been introduced into many European countries. The aim is to improve the coordination of care by focusing on the whole clinical process, building on scientific evidence and involving patients. There is a lack of large-scale and rigorous population-based evaluations, but small-scale studies suggest that DMPs may benefit the process of care and medical outcomes. The evidence on cost–effectiveness is inconclusive. Providers and insurers must make the data they collect available to researchers, and evaluation must become an integral part of chronic disease management.

Integrated care models respond to the fact that chronic diseases can only rarely be treated in isolation. Often patients suffer from several chronic diseases or conditions. These models organize treatment (and prevention) to achieve more integrated services across the whole range of care. The effectiveness of integrated care models is controversial, because the lack of large-scale population-based studies does not allow far-reaching conclusions. Early results suggest that some improvements may be generated but – given the complexity of integrated care – implementation is a key challenge. Future studies must examine implementation problems. It is also not clear which components of integrated care bring about individual improvements. Evidence on cost–effectiveness is also limited: preliminary results are inconclusive.

The third part of the book used this evidence to draw conclusions about the action that policy-makers should take. It also made specific recommendations on how to shape the future. **Pharmaceutical and medical innovations** will continue to play a major part. New pharmaceuticals may lead to better adherence and better quality of life. At the same time, innovative pharmaceuticals will provide a challenge to marketing authorization and reimbursement schemes as well as the evaluation of outcomes.

We have argued that properly applied **financial incentives** can be a powerful means of triggering effective and rapid change in chronic disease management. However, policy-makers need to pay attention to the size of variable compensation or funding and issues relating to goal-setting. Benefits in chronic illness often occur only in the mid or long term, so policy-makers must be aware that the quality of care can often only be improved when providers are sure that their investment is worthwhile. Policy-makers must consider carefully which strategy they are following when aiming to improve continuity of care.

Better **coordination** is critical, because chronic care involves many providers. Research confirms that patients' perception of the quality of care is largely determined by successful coordination. Yet structural, organizational and operational barriers persist. Preliminary conclusions, based on past experience and recent research, suggest that strategic, organizational and operational variables must be taken into account if coordination is to be improved. In particular, policy-makers must recognize that well-organized interests tend to benefit from fragmented care, so reforms aimed at improving coordination should be well prepared, and supported by strong political will. Policy-makers also need to monitor other reforms relating to coordination. They must decide early on whether to depart radically from the current structure, or to build on established norms, institutions and practice. Structurally, policy-makers need to define clearly the responsibilities of the key actors involved. The balance between local autonomy and central authority also needs to be defined. Operationally, sufficient funding is needed to pay for reforms, while at the same time compensation schemes need to be set up that encourage cooperation rather than reinforcing professional separation. Finally, the workforce must be prepared to fulfil its new roles, which means ensuring adequate training, learning and communication.

Another important building block is **ICT**. Theoretical models and some small-scale pilot studies suggest that computerized decision support and data collection can generate many benefits. Using electronic protocols and clinical pathways to support evidence-based medicine is particularly attractive, because it could improve outcomes and reduce medical error. However, the evidence is weak, with only a few rigorous studies on effectiveness and cost–effectiveness.

Experience in many countries has been disappointing: most ICT initiatives run into unexpected difficulties with budget overruns and high costs. If ICT is to meet its potential in chronic disease management, problems of functional interoperability need to be solved through agreement on technical standards. Policy-makers must bring about consensus. Even more important, they must find solutions for translating vast amounts of data into meaningful information for health professionals. They also need to ensure that public concerns regarding data protection are taken into account, and appropriate legislation introduced.

Our work also shows that many strategies and interventions of chronic disease management are not properly **evaluated**. The effectiveness and cost–effectiveness of various prevention and treatment interventions are not well established. Policy-makers are therefore not best equipped to make informed decisions. An important cornerstone for improving knowledge is the development of HTA institutions in several European countries. Policy-makers need better grounded empirical evidence on effectiveness and cost–effectiveness, generated through methodological approaches such as prospective, randomized, controlled evaluation. Policy-makers must ensure that evaluation is an integral part of public programmes. They should also act immediately to make existing data available for research and review, so that an independent and in-depth analysis of effectiveness and cost–effectiveness across different technologies, settings and providers can take place. In the face of increasing globalization of pharmaceutical and health care markets, policy-makers need to ensure that standards for and methods of evidence-based evaluation become internationally accepted. They also need to increase the transparency of procedures and policy decisions.

Finally, we have found that policy-makers do not yet have the information and evidence they need to understand and shape chronic disease management. Future research should concentrate on the issues listed here.

- Evidence based on rigorous research designs needs to be generated for the strategies available to prevent or combat chronic diseases, such as prevention and early detection, new providers and qualifications, DMPs and integrated care. The research should make use of routine population-based data to evaluate key outcomes such as appropriateness, effectiveness and cost–effectiveness, as well as to identify what makes an approach succeed or fail.

- Equally important is that future research examines how specific financial incentives interact with "continuity of care" within different health systems. This question is of fundamental importance for chronic diseases because investment tends to generate health and economic benefits only after 5–10 years have passed. Incentives that lead providers or insurers to make frequent changes may undermine quality of care and cost-containment.

- We suggest that future research should investigate how to translate the vast amounts of data that ICT can store into meaningful information for health professionals.

- Finally, there is a need for international agreement on the acceptability (or even uniformity) of evaluation standards, methods and conduct, as well as for transparency in applying them. There are still no agreed standards and methods, especially regarding the core conflict of fast access to effective technologies and the need for proper, time-consuming comparative evaluation.

References

AcademyHealth (2007). *What is health services research?* Washington, DC, AcademyHealth (http://www.academyhealth.org/about/whatishsr.htm, accessed 25 August 2008).

Åhgren B (2003). Chain of care development in Sweden: Results of a national study. *International Journal of Integrated Care,* 3:e01.

Åhgren B, Axelsson R (2007). Determinants of integrated health care development: Chains of care in Sweden. *International Journal of Health Planning and Management,* 22:145–157.

Alazri M et al. (2006). Patients' experiences of continuity in the care of type 2 diabetes: A focus group study in primary care. *British Journal of General Practice,* 56:488–495.

Aliotta SL et al. (2008). Guided care: A new frontier for adults with chronic conditions. *Professional Case Management,* 13(3):151–158.

Anderson E et al. (2002). NHS walk-in centres and the expanding role of primary care nurses. *Nursing Times,* 98(19):36–37.

Andersson G, Karlberg I (2000). Integrated care for the elderly. The background and effects of the reform of Swedish care of the elderly. *International Journal of Integrated Care,* 1:1–12.

Arun AK (2007). *HPV vaccination – Current status in Europe.* Frost and Sullivan Market Insight (http://www.frost.com/prod/servlet/market-insight-print.pag?docid=100775178, accessed 25 August 2008).

Auld MC (1998). *Wage, alcohol use, and smoking: Simultaneous estimates.* Calgary, Department of Economics, University of Calgary (Discussion Paper No. 98/08).

Averett S, Korenman S (1999). Black-white differences in social and economic consequences of obesity. *International Journal of Obesity*, 23:166–173.

Bakas T et al. (2006). Family caregiving in heart failure. *Nursing Research*, 55(3):180–188.

Bangalore S et al. (2007). Fixed-dose combinations improve medication compliance: A meta-analysis. *American Journal of Medicine*, 120:713–719.

Baron JN, Kreps DM (1999). *Strategic human resources: Frameworks for general managers*. New York, John Wiley & Sons.

Barro R (1996). *Health and economic growth*. Washington, DC, Pan American Health Organization (PAHO) (http://www.paho.org/English/HDP/HDD/barro.pdf, accessed 25 August 2008).

Berndt ER et al. (2000). Lost human capital from early-onset chronic depression. *American Journal of Psychiatry*, 157:940–947.

Beyer M et al. (2006). Wirksamkeit von Disease-Management-Programmen in Deutschland – Probleme der medizinischen Evaluationsforschung anhand eines Studienprotokolls. *Zeitschrift für ärztliche Fortbildung und Qualität im Gesundheitswesen*, 100:355–363.

Bhattacharya J, Bundorf MK (2005). *The incidence of the healthcare costs of obesity*. Cambridge, MA, National Bureau of Economic Research (NBER Working Paper No. 11303).

Bloom BS (2001). Daily regimen and compliance with treatment. *BMJ*, 323:647.

Blum K (2006). Nurse practitioners in eastern Germany. *Health Policy Monitor*, 8, October 2006. University of Auckland, Centre for Health Services Research and Policy (http://www.hpm.org/survey/de/b8/3, accessed 21 August 2009).

Blümel M, Busse R (2009). Disease management programs – Time to evaluate. *Health Policy Monitor*, 13, April 2009. University of Auckland, Centre for Health Services Research and Policy (http://www.hpm.org/survey/de/a13/2, accessed 21 August 2009).

Boaden R et al. (2006). *Evercare evaluation: Final report*. Manchester, National Primary Care Research and Development Centre.

Bodenheimer T, Wagner E, Grumbach K (2002a). Improving primary care for patients with chronic illness. *JAMA*, 288:1775–1779.

Bodenheimer T, Wagner E, Grumbach K (2002b). Improving primary care for patients with chronic illness: The chronic care model. Part 2. *JAMA*, 288:1909–1914.

Boerma W (2006). Coordination and integration in European primary care. In: Saltman R, Rico A, Boerma W (eds). *Primary care in the driver's seat? Organizational reform in European primary care.* Maidenhead, Open University Press:3–21.

Boon H et al. (2004). From parallel practice to integrative health care: A conceptual framework. *BMC Health Services Research,* 4:15.

Bras PL, Duhamel G, Grass E (2006). *Améliorer la prise en charge des maladies chroniques: Les enseignements des expériences étrangères de "disease management".* Paris, Inspection générale des affaires sociales (Rapport RM2006-136P Septembre 2006).

Brown SA, Grimes DE (1995). A meta-analysis of nurse practitioners and nurse midwives in primary care. *Nursing Research,* 44:332–339.

Buchan J, Calman L (2005). *Skill-mix and policy change in the health workforce: Nurses in advanced roles.* Paris, Organisation for Economic Co-operation and Development.

Burton LC, Anderson GF, Kues IW (2004). Using electronic health records to help coordinate care. *Milbank Quarterly,* 82:457–481.

Busse R (2004). Disease management programs in Germany's statutory health insurance system. *Health Affairs (Millwood),* 23(3):56–67.

Busse R, Mays N (2008). Paying for chronic disease care. In: Nolte E, McKee M (eds). *Caring for people with chronic conditions: A health system perspective.* Maidenhead, Open University Press:195–221.

Busse R, Schlette S (2003). *Health policy developments. International trends and analysis. Issue 1.* Gütersloh, Bertelsmann Foundation Publishers.

Busse R, Schlette S (2007). *Health policy developments 7/8. Focus on prevention, health and aging, new health profession.* Gütersloh, Verlag Bertelsmann Stiftung.

Busse R, Zentner A, Schlette S (2006). *Health policy developments 6. Focus on continuity in care, evaluation techniques, IT for health.* Gütersloh, Verlag Bertelsmann Stiftung.

BVA (2008). *Zulassung der Disease Management Programme (DMP) durch das Bundesversicherungsamt.* Bonn, Bundesversicherungsamt (http://www.bundesversicherungsamt.de/nn_1046648/DE/DMP/dmp__node.html?__nnn=true, accessed 23 October 2009).

Calnan M, Hutten J, Tiljak H (2006). The challenge of coordination: The role of primary care professionals in promoting care across the interface. In: Saltman R, Rico A, Boerma W (eds). *Primary care in the driver's seat? Organizational reform in European primary care*. Maidenhead, Open University Press:85–104.

Calnan M et al. (1994). Involvement of the primary health care team in coronary heart disease prevention. *British Journal of General Practice*, 44:224–228.

Campbell S, Reeves D, Kontopantelis E (2007). Quality of primary care in England with the introduction of pay for performance. *New England Journal of Medicine*, 357:181–190.

Campoy F (2005). The Denia Project: Concession for integrated HC. *Health Policy Monitor*, 6, September 2005. University of Auckland, Centre for Health Services Research and Policy (http://www.hpm.org/survey/es/b6/3, accessed 21 August 2009).

Carandang R, Seshadri S, Beiser A (2006). Trends in incidence, lifetime risk, severity, and 30-day mortality of stroke over the past 50 years. *JAMA*, 296:2939–2946.

Casado D (2003). Integrating health and social care. *Health Policy Monitor*, 2, October 2003. University of Auckland, Centre for Health Services Research and Policy (http://www.hpm.org/survey/es/b2/4, accessed 21 August 2009).

Cawley J (2004). The impact of obesity on wages. *Journal of Human Resources*, 32:451–474.

Cawley J (2007). The cost–effectiveness of programs to prevent or reduce obesity: The state of the literature and a future research agenda. *Archives of Pediatrics & Adolescent Medicine*, 161:611–614.

Chobanian AV et al. (2003). The seventh report of the joint national committee on prevention, detection, evaluation, and treatment of high blood pressure: The JNC 7 report. *JAMA*, 289:2560–2572.

CHSRP (2005). Cancer control action plan. *Health Policy Monitor*, 5, April 2005. University of Auckland, Centre for Health Services Research and Policy (http://www.hpm.org/survey/nz/a5/3, accessed 21 August 2009).

CHSRP (2006). Development of nurse practitioners. *Health Policy Monitor*, 8, October 2006. University of Auckland, Centre for Health Services Research and Policy (http://www.hpm.org/survey/nz/a8/4, accessed 21 August 2009).

CHSRP et al. (2006). An inter-sectoral approach to diabetes. *Health Policy Monitor*, 7, April 2006. University of Auckland, Centre for Health Services Research and Policy (http://www.hpm.org/survey/nz/a7/3, accessed 21 August 2009).

Claxton AJ, Cramer J, Pierce C (2001). A systematic review of the associations between dose regimens and medication compliance. *Clinical Therapeutics,* 23(8):1296–1310.

Cline C (2002). Nurse-led clinics for heart failure in Sweden – Doing the right thing? *European Journal of Heart Failure,* 4:393–394.

Coiera E (2003). Clinical decision support systems. In: Coiera E. *Guide to health informatics.* 2nd edition. London, Arnold:331–345.

Coile C (2003). *Health shocks and couples' labor supply decisions.* Chestnut Hill, MA, Center for Retirement Research at Boston College (Working Paper No. 2003-08).

Connor CA, Wright CC, Fegan CD (2002). The safety and effectiveness of a nurse-led anticoagulant service. *Journal of Advanced Nursing,* 38:407–415.

Couffinhal A (2003). Drug price liberalization. *Health Policy Monitor,* 1, May 2003. University of Auckland, Centre for Health Services Research and Policy (http://www.hpm.org/survey/fr/a1/2, accessed 25 August 2008).

Craig BM, Tseng DS (2002). Cost effectiveness of gastric bypass for severe obesity. *American Journal of Medicine,* 113:491–498.

Department of Health (2004). *The NHS improvement plan. Putting people at the heart of public services.* London, Department of Health.

Disease Control Priorities Project (2007). *Cost effective interventions.* Washington, DC, Disease Control Priorities Project (http://www.dcp2.org/page/main/BrowseInterventions.html, accessed 21 August 2009).

Dubois C-A, Singh D, Jiwani I (2008). The human resource challenge in chronic care. In: Nolte E, McKee M (eds). *Caring for people with chronic conditions: A health system perspective.* Maidenhead, Open University Press:143–171.

Durand-Zaleski I, Obrecht O (2008). France. In: Knai C, Nolte E, McKee M (eds) *Managing chronic conditions: Experience in eight countries.* Copenhagen, WHO Regional Office for Europe, on behalf of the European Observatory on Health Systems and Policies:55–73.

Dwyer DS, Mitchell OS (1999). Health problems as determinants of retirement: Are self-rated measures endogenous? *Journal of Health Economics,* 18:173–193.

Eastman R et al. (1997). Models of complications of NIDDM. II. Analysis of the health benefits and cost–effectiveness of treating NIDDM with the goal of normoglycaemia. *Diabetes Care,* 20:685–686.

Eccles M, McColl E, Steen N (2002). Effect of computerised evidence-based guidelines on management of asthma and angina in adults in primary care: Cluster randomised controlled trial. *BMJ,* 325:1–7.

Edwards BK et al. (2002). Annual report to the nation on the status of cancer, 1973–1999, featuring implications of age and aging on US cancer burden. *Cancer,* 94(10):2766–2792.

Engström S, Foldevi M, Borgquist L (2001). Is general practice effective? A systematic literature review. *Scandinavian Journal of Primary Health Care,* 19:131–144.

Epping-Jordan J et al. (2004). Improving the quality of care for chronic conditions. *Quality and Safety in Health Care,* 13:299–305.

Ernst M, Moolchan E, Robinson M (2001). Behavioural and neural consequences of prenatal exposure to nicotine. *Journal of the American Academy of Child Adolescent Psychiatry,* 40:630–641.

European Commission (2000). *EURODIET Core Report – Nutrition & Diet for Healthy Lifestyles in Europe, Science & Policy Implications.* Crete, European Commission and University of Crete School of Medicine.

European Commission (2004). *Building a European health survey system: improving information on self-perceived morbidity and chronic conditions.* Brussels, European Commission Working Party Morbidity and Mortality.

European Commission (2008). *Communication from the Commission to the European Parliament, the Council, the European Economic and Social Committee and the Committee of the Regions on telemedicine for the benefit of patients, healthcare systems and society.* Brussels, European Commission (http://eur-lex. europa.eu/LexUriServ/LexUriServ.do?uri=COM:2008:0689:FIN:EN:PDF, accessed 21 August 2009).

European Commission (2009). *i2010 – A European information society for growth and employment.* Brussels, European Commission (http://ec.europa. eu/information_society/eeurope/i2010/index_en.htm, accessed 21 August 2009).

European Network for Smoking Prevention (2004). *Effective tobacco control in 28 European countries.* Brussels, European Network for Smoking Prevention (www.ensp.org/files/effectivefinal2.pdf, accessed 25 August 2008).

Evans D (1996). *A stakeholder analysis of developments at the primary and secondary care interface.* Southampton, Institute for Health Policy Studies, University of Southampton.

Ferri C et al. (2005). Global prevalence of dementia: A Delphi consensus study. *Lancet*, 366:2112–2117.

Fielding JE (1996). Getting smarter and maybe wiser. *American Journal of Health Promotion*, 11:109–111.

Fireman B, Bartlett J, Selby J (2004). Can disease management reduce health care costs by improving quality? *Health Affairs*, 23(6):63–75.

Freeman G, Woloshynowych M, Baker R (2007). *Continuity of care 2006: What have we learned since 2000 and what are policy imperatives now?* London, National Co-ordinating Centre for NHS Service Delivery and Organisation Research and Development.

Frossard M et al. (2002). *Providing integrated health and social care for older persons in France – An old idea with a great future.* Paris, Union nationale interfédérale des œuvres et organismes privés sanitaires et sociaux.

Gallagher-Thompson D, Coon DW (2007). Evidence-based psychological treatments for distress in family caregivers of older adults. *Psychology and Aging*, 22(1):37–51.

Gannon B, Nolan B (2004). Disability and labor force participation in Ireland. *The Economic and Social Review*, 35.135–155.

Garg AX, Adhikari NK, McDonald H (2005). Effects of computerized clinical decision support systems on practitioner performance and patient outcomes: A systematic review. *JAMA*, 293:1223–1238.

Gertler P, Levine DI, Ames A (2004). Schooling and parental death. *The Review of Economics and Statistics*, 86:211–225.

Gervas J, Perez-Fernandez M, Starfield BH (1994). Primary care, financing and gatekeeping in western Europe. *Family Practice*, 11:307–317.

Ginsburg GS, McCarthy J (2001). Personalized medicine: Revolutionizing drug discovery and patient care. *Trends in Biotechnology*, 19:491–496.

Glasgow N et al. (2008). Australia. In: Knai C, Nolte E, McKee M (eds). *Managing chronic conditions: Experience in eight countries.* Copenhagen, WHO Regional Office for Europe, on behalf of the European Observatory on Health Systems and Policies:131–160.

Goodwin N et al. (2004). *Managing across diverse networks of care: Lessons from other sectors.* London, National Co-ordinating Centre for NHS Service Delivery and Organisation Research and Development.

Gortmaker SL et al. (1993). Social and economic consequences of overweight in adolescence and young adulthood. *New England Journal of Medicine,* 329:1008–1012.

Grant JS et al. (2004). Caregiving problems and feelings experienced by family caregivers of stroke survivors the first month after discharge. *International Journal of Rehabilitation Research,* 27(2):105–111.

Gravelle H et al. (2007). Impact of case management (Evercare) on frail elderly patients: Controlled before and after analysis of quantitative outcome data. *BMJ,* 334:31–34.

Greenberger H, Litwin H (2003). Can burdened caregivers be effective facilitators of elder care-recipient health care? *Journal of Advanced Nursing,* 41(4):332–341.

Griffiths C, Foster G, Barnes N (2004). Specialist nurse intervention to reduce unscheduled asthma care in a deprived multiethnic area: The east London randomized controlled trial for high risk asthma (ELECTRA). *BMJ,* 328:144.

Gross R, Tabenkin H, Brammli-Greenberg S (2000). Who needs a gatekeeper? Patients' views of the role of the primary care physician. *Family Practice,* 17:222–229.

Grundmeyer HGLM (1996). General practitioner and specialist: Why do they communicate so badly? *European Journal of General Practice,* 2:53–54.

Haas M (2005). NSW chronic care collaboratives. *Health Policy Monitor,* 6, October 2005. University of Auckland, Centre for Health Services Research and Policy (http://www.hpm.org/survey/au/a6/4, accessed 25 August 2008).

Haley WE et al. (2003). Predictors of depression and life satisfaction among spousal caregivers in hospice: Application of a stress process model. *Journal of Palliative Medicine,* 6(2):215–224.

Haskins KM, Ransford HE (1999). The relationship between weight and career payoffs among women. *Sociological Forum,* 14:295–318.

Hayden-Wade HA et al. (2005). Prevalence, characteristics, and correlates of teasing experiences among overweight children vs. non-overweight peers. *Obesity Research,* 13:1381–1392.

Hendy J et al. (2005). Challenges to implementing the national programme for information technology (NPfIT): A qualitative study. *BMJ,* 331:331–336.

Hofmarcher M, Oxley H, Rusticelli E (2007). *Improved health system performance through better care coordination.* Paris, Organisation for Economic Co-operation and Development.

Horrocks S, Anderson E, Salisbury C (2002). Systematic review of whether nurse practitioners working in primary care can provide equivalent care to doctors. *BMJ,* 324:819–823.

Hroscikoski M et al. (2006). Challenges of change: A qualitative study of chronic care model implementation. *Annals of Family Medicine,* 4:317–326.

Hunter D, Fairfield G (1997). Managed care: Disease management. *BMJ,* 315:50–53.

James WPT et al. (2004). Overweight and obesity (high body mass index). In: Ezzati M et al. *Comparative quantification of health risks: Global and regional burden of disease attributable to selected major risk factors.* Geneva, World Health Organization (http://www.who.int/publications/cra, accessed 25 August 2008).

Jamison D (2006). Investing in health. In: Jamison D et al. *Disease control priorities in developing countries.* 2nd edition. New York, Oxford University Press:3–36.

Jha P, Chaloupka F (2000). *Tobacco control in developing countries.* Oxford, Oxford University Press.

Jha P et al. (2006). Tobacco addiction. In: Jamison D et al. *Disease control priorities in developing countries.* 2nd edition. New York, Oxford University Press:869–886.

Jiménez-Martín S, Labeaga JM, Martínez Granado M (1999). *Health status and retirement decisions for older European couples.* IRISS Working Paper No. 1999-01. Luxembourg, Integrated Research Infrastructure in Social Sciences.

Joos S, Rosemann T, Heiderhoff M (2005). ELSID-Diabetes study – Evaluation of a large scale implementation of disease management programmes for patients with type 2 diabetes. Rationale design and conduct: A study protocol. *BMC Public Health,* 5:99.

Kane R et al. (2004). Patterns of utilization for the Minnesota senior health options program. *Journal of the American Geriatrics Society,* 52:2039–2044.

Karlberg I (2008). Sweden. In: Knai C, Nolte E, McKee M (eds). *Managing chronic conditions: Experience in eight countries.* Copenhagen, WHO Regional Office for Europe, on behalf of the European Observatory on Health Systems and Policies:115–130.

Kerr E, Fleming B (2007). Making performance indicators work: Experiences of US Veterans Health Administration. *BMJ*, 335:971–973.

Kessler R (2007). The global burden of anxiety and mood disorders: Putting the European study of epidemiology of mental disorders (ESEMeD) findings into perspective. *Journal of Clinical Psychiatry*, 68(Suppl. 2):10–19.

Kheir NM et al. (2004). Health-related quality of life measurement in pharmaceutical care. Targeting an outcome that matters. *Pharmacy World and Science*, 26:125–128.

Kinnersley P, Anderson E, Parry K (2000). Randomised controlled trial of nurse practitioner versus general practitioner care for patients requesting "same day" consultations in primary care. *BMJ*, 320:1043–1048.

Kinsella K, Phillips D (2005). Global aging: The challenge of success. *Population Bulletin*, 60:5–42.

Kraut A et al. (2001). Impact of diabetes on employment and income in Manitoba, Canada. *Diabetes Care*, 24:64–68.

Latner JD, Stunkard, AJ (2003). Getting worse: The stigmatisation of obese children. *Obesity Research*, 11:452–456.

Leatherman S, Berwick D, Iles D (2003). The business case for quality: Case studies and an analysis. *Health Affairs*, 22(2):17–30.

Lee Y (1999). *Wage effects of drinking and smoking: An analysis using Australian twins data*. Crawley, Department of Economics, University of Western Australia (Working Paper No. 99–22).

Lester WT et al. (2006). Randomized controlled trial of an informatics-based intervention to increase statin prescription for secondary prevention of coronary disease. *Journal of General Internal Medicine*, 21:22–29.

Leutz W (1999). Five laws for integrating medical and social services: Lessons from the United States and the United Kingdom. *Milbank Quarterly*, 77:77–110.

Levine C (1999). Home sweet hospital: The nature and limits of private responsibilities for home health care. *Journal of Aging and Health*, 11(3): 341–359.

Levine PB, Gustafson TA, Valenchik AD (1997). More bad news for smokers? The effects of cigarette smoking on wages. *Industrial and Labor Relations Review*, 50:493–509.

Lewis LD (2005). Personalized drug therapy; the genome, the chip and the physician. *British Journal of Clinical Pharmacology*, 60:1–4.

Lindholm C, Burstrom B, Diderichsen F (2001). Does chronic illness cause adverse social and economic consequences among Swedes? *Scandinavian Journal of Public Health*, 29:63–70.

Lohr KN, Steinwachs DM (2002). Health services research: An evolving definition of the field. *Health Services Research*, 37:15–17.

Lopez AD et al. (2006) *Global burden of disease and risk factors*. New York, Oxford University Press and World Bank.

McAlister FA et al. (2001a). A systematic review of randomized trials of disease management programmes in heart failure. *American Journal of Medicine*, 110:378–384.

McAlister FA et al. (2001b). Randomized trials of secondary prevention programmes in coronary heart disease: A systematic review. *BMJ*, 323:9575–9962.

McCowan C, Neville RG, Ricketts IW (2001). Lessons from a randomized controlled trial designed to evaluate computer decision support software to improve the management of asthma. *Medical Informatics and the Internet in Medicine*, 26:191–201.

McCusker J et al. (2007). Major depression among medically ill elders contributes to sustained poor mental health in their informal caregivers. *Age and Ageing*, 36(4):400–406.

McGarry K (2002). *Health and retirement: Do changes in health affect retirement expectations?* Cambridge, MA, National Bureau of Economic Research (NBER Working Paper No. 9317).

McIntosh T (2006). Provincial health human resource plans. *Health Policy Monitor*, 7, April 2006. University of Auckland, Centre for Health Services Research and Policy (http://www.hpm.org/survey/ca/a7/2, accessed 21 August 2009).

McKee M, Healy J (2002). Réorganisation des systèmes hospitaliers: leçons tirées de l'Europe de l'Ouest. *Revue Médicale de l'Assurance Maladie*, 33:31–36.

Maetzel A et al. (2003). Economic evaluation of orlistat in overweight and obese patients with type 2 diabetes mellitus. *Pharmacoeconomics*, 21:501–512.

Manotti C, Moia M, Palareti G (2001). Effect of computer-aided management on the quality of treatment in anticoagulated patients: A prospective, randomized, multicenter trial of APROAT (automated program for oral anticoagulant treatment). *Haematologica*, 86:1060–1070.

Martin DP et al. (1989). Effect of a gatekeeper plan on health services use and charges: A randomized trial. *American Journal of Public Health,* 79(12): 1628–1632.

Mathers CD, Loncar D (2005). *Updated projections of global mortality and burden of disease, 2002–2030: Data sources, methods and results.* Geneva, World Health Organization (Evidence and Information for Policy Working Paper). (http://www.who.int/healthinfo/statistics/bod_projections2030_paper.pdf, accessed 21 August 2009).

Mathers CD et al. (2003). *The global burden of disease in 2002: Data sources, methods and results.* Geneva, World Health Organization (GPE discussion paper No. 54). (http://www.who.int/healthinfo/paper54.pdf, accessed 21 August 2009).

Mattke S, Seid M, Sai M (2007). Evidence for the effect of disease management: Is US$ 1 billion a year a good investment? *American Journal of Managed Care,* 13:670–676.

Messecar D, Powers BA, Nagel CL (2008). The Family Preferences Index: helping family members who want to participate in the care of a hospitalized older adult. *American Journal of Nursing,* 108(9):52–59.

Meyer TJ et al. (1996). Randomized controlled trial of residents as gatekeepers. *Archives of Internal Medicine:*156(21):2483–2487.

Mitra A (2001). Effects of physical attributes on the wages of males and females. *Applied Economics Letters,* 8:731–735.

Murray MD, Harris LE, Overhage JM (2004). Failure of computerized treatment suggestions to improve health outcomes of outpatients with uncomplicated hypertension: Results of a randomized controlled trial. *Pharmacotherapy,* 24:324–337.

Narayan Venkat KM et al. (2006). Diabetes: The pandemic and potential solutions. In: Jamison D et al. *Disease control priorities in developing countries.* 2nd edition. New York, Oxford University Press:591–604.

Naudin F, Sermet C (2003). Drug delisting and reduced reimbursement. *Health Policy Monitor,* 2, October 2003. University of Auckland, Centre for Health Services Research and Policy (http://www.hpm.org/survey/fr/a2/1, accessed 21 August 2009).

Ng Y, Jacobs P, Johnson JA (2001). Productivity losses associated with diabetes in the US. *Diabetes Care,* 24:257–261.

Nolte E, Mckee M (2008). Integration and chronic care: A review. In: Nolte E, McKee M (eds). *Caring for people with chronic conditions: A health system perspective*. Maidenhead, Open University Press:64–91.

Norris SL et al. (2002). The effectiveness of disease and case management for people with diabetes. *American Journal of Preventive Medicine,* 22(4S):15–38.

Novotny TE (2008). Preventing chronic disease: Everybody's business. In: Nolte E, McKee M (eds). *Caring for people with chronic conditions: A health system perspective.* Maidenhead, Open University Press:92–115.

O'Connor AM, Stacey D, Entwistle V (2003). Decision aids can help people take an active role in making informed decisions about healthcare options. *Cochrane Database of Systematic Reviews,* Issue 1. Art. No. CD001431. DOI: 10.1002/14651858.CD001431.

O'Connor PJ, Lauren Crain A, Rush WA (2005). Impact of an electronic medical record on diabetes quality of care. *Annals of Family Medicine,* 4: 300–306.

Ofman JJ, Badamgarav E, Henning JM (2004). Does disease management improve clinical and economic outcomes in patients with chronic diseases? A systematic review. *American Journal of Medicine,* 117.182–192.

Oliver A (2005). Screening for bowel cancer. *Health Policy Monitor,* 5, March 2005. University of Auckland, Centre for Health Services Research and Policy (http.//www.hpm.org/survey/uk/a5/3, accessed 21 August 2009).

Ose D et al. (2009). Impact of primary care-based disease management on the health-related quality of life in patients with type 2 diabetes and co-morbidity. *Diabetes Care* (published ahead of print) (http://care.diabetesjournals. org/content/early/2009/06/05/dc08-2223.full.pdf+html, accessed 18 August 2009).

Øvretveit J (1998). *Evaluating health interventions.* Maidenhead, Open University Press.

Pelikan JM, Nowak P (1998). Concepts on the topic "Quality in health care". In: Federal Ministry of Labour, Health and Social Affairs (ed.). *Quality in health care.* Vienna, Conference Report of Meeting of European Health Ministries on Quality in Health Care.

Pelkowski JM, Berger MC (2004). The impact of health on employment, wages, and hours worked over the life-cycle. *The Quarterly Review of Economics and Finance,* 44:102–121.

Petermann F (1996). *Lebensqualität und chronische Krankheit.* Munich, Dustri-Verlag.

Petersen L et al. (2006). Does pay-for-performance improve the quality of health care? *Annals of Internal Medicine,* 145:265–272.

Piatt G et al. (2006). Translating the chronic care model into the community. Results from a randomized controlled trial of a multifaceted diabetes care intervention. *Diabetes Care,* 29:811–817.

Pilnick A, Dingwall R, Starkey K (2001). Disease management: Definitions, difficulties and future directions. *Bulletin of the World Health Organization,* 79:755–763.

Plaza V, Cobos A, Ignacio-Garcia JM (2005). Cost–effectiveness of an intervention based on the global initiative for asthma (GINA) recommendations using a computerized clinical decision support system: A physician's randomized trial. *Medicina Clinicia,* 124(6):201–206.

Plochg T, Klazinga N (2002). Community-based integrated care: Myth or must? *International Journal for Quality in Health Care,* 14:91–101.

Pomerleau J, Knai C, Nolte E (2008). The burden of chronic disease in Europe. In: Nolte E, McKee M (eds). *Caring for people with chronic conditions: A health system perspective.* Maidenhead, Open University Press:15–42.

Preston C et al. (1999). Left in limbo: Patients' views on care across the primary/secondary interface. *Quality in Health Care,* 8:16–21.

Pronk NP et al. (2004). The association between work performance and physical activity, cardiorespiratory fitness, and obesity. *Journal of Occupational and Environmental Medicine,* 46:19–25.

Prosser LA et al. (2000). Cost–effectiveness of cholesterol-lowering therapies according to selected patient characteristics. *Annals of Internal Medicine,* 132:769–779.

Rodgers A et al. (2006). The growing burden of risk from high blood pressure, cholesterol and bodyweight. In: Jamison D et al. *Disease control priorities in developing countries.* 2nd edition. New York, Oxford University Press: 851–868.

Roland M (2004). Linking physicians' pay to the quality of care – A major experiment in the United Kingdom. *New England Journal of Medicine,* 351:1448–1454.

Rollman BL, Hanusa BH, Lowe HJ (2002). A randomized trial using computerized decision support to improve treatment of major depression in primary care. *Journal of General Internal Medicine,* 17:493–503.

Rosemann T, Joest K, Koerner T (2006). How can the practice nurse be more involved in the care of the chronically ill? The perspectives of GPs, patients and practice nurses. *BMC Family Practice*, 7:14.

Roux L et al. (2006). Economic evaluation of weight loss interventions in overweight and obese women. *Obesity*, 14:1093–1106.

Salisbury C (2004). Does advanced access work for patients and practices? *British Journal of General Practice*, 54:330–331.

Sandier S, Paris V, Polton D (2004). *Health care systems in transition: France*. Copenhagen, WHO Regional Office for Europe, on behalf of the European Observatory on Health Systems and Policies.

Sargent J, Blanchflower DG (1994). Obesity and stature in adolescence and earnings in young adulthood: Analysis of a British birth cohort. *Archives of Pediatrics and Adolescent Medicine*, 148:681–687.

Sargent P et al. (2007). Patient and carer perceptions of case management for long-term conditions. *Health and Social Care in the Community*, 15:511–519.

Sarlio-Lahteenkorva S, Lahelma E (1999). The association of body mass index with social and economic disadvantage in women and men. *International Journal of Epidemiology*, 28:445–449.

Sawicki PT et al. (2006). *Kontrollierte Evaluation der Effekte von Disease-Management-Programmen für Patienten mit Diabetes mellitus Typ 2 und Patienten mit koronarer Herzkrankheit. Teil: Diabetes Mellitus Typ 2*. Köln, DIeM- Institut für evidenzbasierte Medizin.

Schang L (2009) Morbidity-based risk structure compensation. *Health Policy Monitor*, 13, April 2009. University of Auckland, Centre for Health Services Research and Policy (http://www.hpm.org/survey/de/b13/1, accessed 21 August 2009).

Schiøtz M, Frølich A, Krasnik A (2008). Denmark. In: Knai C, Nolte E, McKee M (eds). *Managing chronic conditions: Experience in eight countries*. Copenhagen, WHO Regional Office for Europe, on behalf of the European Observatory on Health Systems and Policies:15–28.

Schoen C, Osborn R, Doty M (2007). Toward higher-performance health systems: Adult's health care experiences in seven countries. *Health Affairs*, 26: w717–w734.

Schumacher K, Beck CA, Marren JM (2006). Family caregivers: Caring for older adults, working with their families. *American Journal of Nursing*, 106(8):40–49.

Scott JT et al. (2005). Kaiser Permanente's experience of implementing an electronic medical record: A qualitative study. *BMJ*, 331:1313–1316.

Serxner SA, Gold DB, Bultman KK (2001). The impact of behavioral health risks on worker absenteeism. *Journal of Occupational and Environmental Medicine*, 43:347–354.

Shane R (2007). Management of chronic diseases in the 21st century: The emerging role of specialty pharmacies. *American Journal of Health-System Pharmacy*, 64:2382–2385.

Shum C, Humphreys A, Wheeler D (2000). Nurse management of patients with minor illnesses in general practice: Multicentre, randomised controlled trial. *BMJ*, 320:1038–1043.

Shurin AB, Nabel EG (2008). Pharmacogenomics – Ready for prime time? *New England Journal of Medicine*, 358:1061–1063.

Sidorov J et al. (2002). Does diabetes disease management save money and improve outcomes? A report of simultaneous short-term savings and quality improvement associated with a health maintenance organization – Sponsored disease management program among patients fulfilling health employer data and information set criteria. *Diabetes Care*, 25:684–689.

Siering U (2008). Germany. In: Knai C, Nolte E, McKee, M (eds). *Managing chronic conditions: Experience in eight countries*. Copenhagen, WHO Regional Office for Europe, on behalf of the European Observatory on Health Systems and Policies:75–96.

Simon GE et al. (2000). Recovery from depression, work productivity, and health care costs among primary care patients. *General Hospital Psychiatry*, 22:153–162.

Singh D (2005a). *Transforming chronic care*. Birmingham, University of Birmingham and Surrey and Sussex PCT Alliance.

Singh D (2005b). *Which staff improve care for people with long-term conditions? A rapid review of the literature*. Birmingham, University of Birmingham and NHS Modernisation Agency.

Singh D (2008). *How can chronic disease management programmes operate across care settings and providers?* Copenhagen, WHO Regional Office for Europe, on behalf of the European Observatory on Health Systems and Policies.

Singh D, Fahey D (2008). England. In: Knai C, Nolte E, McKee M (eds). *Managing chronic conditions: Experience in eight countries*. Copenhagen, WHO Regional Office for Europe, on behalf of the European Observatory on Health Systems and Policies:29–54.

Singh D, Ham C (2006). *Improving care for people with long-term conditions. A review of UK and international frameworks.* Birmingham, University of Birmingham, NHS Institute for Innovation and Improvement.

Sloan FA et al. (2004). *The price of smoking.* Cambridge, MA, and London, MIT Press.

Smith B et al. (2001). Home care by outreach nursing for chronic obstructive pulmonary disease. *Cochrane Database of Systematic Reviews,* 3:CD000994.

Smith S, Bury G, O'Leary M (2004). The North Dublin randomized controlled trial of structured diabetes shared care. *Family Practice,* 21:39–45.

Smith P, York N (2004). Quality incentives: The case of UK general practitioners. *Health Affairs,* 23(3):112–118.

Solberg L et al. (2006). Care quality and implementation of the chronic care model: A quantitative study. *Annals of Family Medicine,* 4:310–316.

Sorenson C et al. (2008). *How can the impact of health technology assessments be enhanced?* Copenhagen, WHO Regional Office for Europe, on behalf of the European Observatory on Health Systems and Policies (http://www.euro.who. int/document/hsm/2_hsc08_ePB_5.pdf, accessed 21 August 2009).

Starfield B, Shi L, Macinko J (2005). Contribution of primary care to health systems and health. *Milbank Quarterly,* 83.457–502.

Steuten LMG et al. (2002). Participation of general practitioners in disease management: Experiences from the Netherlands. *International Journal of Integrated Care,* 2:e24.

Stromberg A, Martensson J, Fridlund B (2003). Nurse-led heart failure clinics improve survival and self-care behaviour in patients with heart failure: Results from a prospective, randomised trial. European *Heart Journal,* 24:1014–1023.

Suhrcke M, Urban D (2006). *Are cardiovascular diseases bad for economic growth?* Copenhagen, WHO Regional Office for Europe.

Suhrcke M, Fahey DK, McKee M (2008). Economic aspects of chronic disease and chronic disease management. In: Nolte E, McKee M (eds). *Caring for people with chronic conditions: A health system perspective.* Maidenhead, Open University Press:43–63.

Suhrcke M, Rocco L, McKee M (2007a). *Health: A vital investment for economic development in eastern Europe and central Asia.* Copenhagen, WHO Regional Office for Europe on behalf of the European Observatory on Health Systems and Policies.

Suhrcke M, Rocco L, McKee M (2007b). *Economic consequences of noncommunicable diseases and injuries in the Russian Federation.* Copenhagen, WHO Regional Office for Europe on behalf of the European Observatory on Health Systems and Policies.

Suhrcke M et al. (2005). *The contribution of health to the economy in the European Union.* Brussels, European Commission.

Suhrcke M et al. (2006). *Chronic disease: An economic perspective* (with annex). London, Oxford Health Alliance (http://www.oxha.org/knowledge/publications/oxha-chronic-disease-an-economic-perspective.pdf and http://www.oxha.org/knowledge/publications/annextoeconomicsreport.pdf, accessed 4 December 2009).

Szecsenyi J (2008). *Pressegespräch zu den Ergebnissen der ELSID-Studie am 12.08.2008 in Berlin.* Berlin, AOK-Bundesverband (http://www.aok-prodialog.de/inc_ges/download/dl.php/wl/dmp/imperia/md/content/aokbundesverband/dokumente/pdf/presse/statement_szecsenyi_elsid_120808.pdf, accessed 10 February 2010).

Szecsenyi J et al. (2008). German diabetes disease management programs are appropriate to restructure care according to the chronic care model. *Diabetes Care,* 31:1150–1154.

Tierney WM, Overhage JM, Murray MD (2005). Can computer-generated evidence-based care suggestions enhance evidence-based management of asthma and chronic obstructive pulmonary disease? A randomized controlled trial. *Health Services Research,* 40:311–315.

Torgerson, RC (2005a) Interprofessional education. *Health Policy Monitor,* 6, October 2005. University of Auckland, Centre for Health Services Research and Policy (http://www.hpm.org/survey/ca/a6/1, accessed 21 August 2009).

Torgerson, RC (2005b) Ontario's local health integration networks. *Health Policy Monitor,* 6, October 2005. University of Auckland, Centre for Health Services Research and Policy (http://www.hpm.org/survey/ca/a6/2, accessed 25 August 2008).

Tucker LA, Friedman GM (1998). Obesity and absenteeism: An epidemiologic study of 10,825 employed adults. *American Journal of Health Promotion,* 12:202–207.

Tuffs A (2004). Germany plans to introduce electronic health card. *BMJ,* 329:131.

Tuffs A (2006). Introduction of Germany's electronic health cards is delayed. *BMJ,* 332:72.

Turner D, Tarrant C, Windridge K (2007). Do patients value continuity of care in general practice? An investigation using stated preference discrete choice experiments. *Journal of Health Services Research and Policy,* 12:132–137.

UnitedHealth Europe (2005). *Assessment of the Evercare programme in England 2003–2004.* London, UnitedHealth.

Van der Linden BA, Spreeuwenberg C, Schrijvers AJP (2001). Integration of care in the Netherlands: The development of transmural care since 1994. *Health Policy,* 55:111–120.

Van der Maas P, Mackenbach J (1999). *Volksgezondheid en gezondheidszorg [Public health and health care].* Maarssen, Elsevier/Bunge.

Van Dijk JK (2003). Nurse practitioner update. *Health Policy Monitor,* 2, December 2003. University of Auckland, Centre for Health Services Research and Policy (http://www.hpm.org/survey/nl/b2/1, accessed 21 August 2009).

Van Dulmen S et al. (2007). Patient adherence to medical treatment: A review of reviews. *BMC Health Services Research,* 7:55.

Van Ginneken E, Busse R, Gericke CA (2008). Universal private health insurance in the Netherlands: The first year. *Journal of Management & Marketing in Healthcare,* 1:139–153.

Van Gool K (2005). PBAC processes. *Health Policy Monitor,* 5, April 2005. University of Auckland, Centre for Health Services Research and Policy (http://www.hpm.org/survey/au/a5/4, accessed 21 August 2009).

Van Lente EJ, Willenborg P, Egger B (2008). Auswirkungen der Disease-Management-Programme auf die Versorgung chronisch kranker Patienten in Deutschland – eine Zwischenbilanz. *Gesundheits- und Sozialpolitik,* 62(3):10 18.

Van Ours JC (2004). A pint a day raises a man's pay; but smoking blows that gain away. *Journal of Health Economics,* 23:863–886.

Velasco Garrido M, Busse R, Hisashige A (2003). *Are disease management programmes (DMPs) effective in improving quality of care for people with chronic conditions?* Copenhagen, WHO Regional Office for Europe (Health Evidence Network report) (http://www.euro.who.int/document/e82974.pdf, accessed 25 August 2008).

Velasco-Garrido M et al. (eds) (2008). *Health technology assessment and health policy-making in Europe: Current status, challenges and potential.* Copenhagen, WHO Regional Office for Europe, on behalf of the European Observatory on Health Systems and Policies (http://www.euro.who.int/Document/E91922.pdf, accessed 21 August 2009).

Villagra VG, Ahmed T (2004). Effectiveness of a disease management program for patients with diabetes. *Health Affairs,* 23(4):255–266.

Vrijhoef HJ, Diederiks JP, Spreeuwenberg C (2000). Effects on quality of care for patients with NIDDM or COPD when the specialised nurse has a central role: A literature review. *Patient Education and Counselling,* 41:243–250.

Vrijhoef HJ et al. (2001). Substitution model with central role for nurse specialist is justified in the care for stable type 2 diabetic outpatients. *Journal of Advanced Nursing,* 36:546–555.

Vrijhoef HJ et al. (2003). Undiagnosed patients and patients at risk for COPD in primary health care: Early detection with the support of non-physicians. *Journal of Clinical Nursing,* 12:366–373.

Wagner E et al. (1999). A survey of leading chronic disease management programs: Are they consistent with the literature? *Managed Care Quarterly,* 7:56–66.

Wald NJ, Law MR (2003). A strategy to reduce cardiovascular disease by more than 80%. *BMJ,* 326:1419.

Wang LY et al. (2003). Economic analysis of a school-based obesity prevention program. *Obesity Research,* 11:1313–1324.

Wang Y et al. (2006). Practice size and quality attainment under the new GMS contract: A cross-sectional analysis. *British Journal of General Practice,* 56: 830–835.

Weingarten SR, Henning JM, Badamgarav E (2002). Interventions used in disease management programmes for patients with chronic illness – Which ones work? Meta-analysis of published reports. *BMJ,* 325:925.

WHO (1991). *Assessment of quality of life in health care: A working party report.* Geneva, World Health Organization.

WHO (2002). *The world health report 2002 – Reducing risks, promoting healthy life.* Geneva, World Health Organization (http://www.who.int/whr/2002/en/, accessed August 25, 2008).

WHO (2003). *Adherence to long-term therapies: Evidence for action.* Geneva, World Health Organization (http://www.who.int/chp/knowledge/publications/ adherence full_report.pdf, accessed 17 August 2008).

WHO (2005). *Preventing chronic diseases: A vital investment.* Geneva, World Health Organization (http://www.who.int/chp/chronic_disease_report/full_ report.pdf, accessed 25 August 2008).

WHO (2008a). *The global burden of disease: 2004 update.* Geneva, World Health Organization (http://www.who.int/entity/healthinfo/global_burden_disease/GBD_report_2004update_full.pdf, accessed 12 January 2010).

WHO (2008b). *Health statistics and health information systems. Projections of mortality and burden of disease, 2004-2030.* Geneva, World Health Organization (http://www.who.int/healthinfo/global_burden_disease/projections/en/index.html, accessed 12 January 2010).

WHO (2009). *WHO statistical information system. Age-standardized death rates and DALYs, by cause, and Member State, 2004.* Geneva, World Health Organization (http://www.who.int/entity/healthinfo/global_burden_disease/gbddeathdalycountryestimates2004.xls, accessed 12 January 2010).

WHO Regional Office for Europe (2004). *A strategy to prevent chronic disease in Europe: A focus on public health action: The CINDI vision.* Copenhagen, WHO Regional Office for Europe (http://www.euro.who.int/document/e83057.pdf, accessed 25 August 2008).

Wilking N, Jönsson B (2005). *A pan-European comparison regarding patient access to cancer drugs.* Stockholm, Karolinska Institutet in collaboration with Stockholm School of Economics (http://ki.se/content/1/c4/33/52/Cancer_Report.pdf, accessed 25 August 2008).

Wilkins VM, Bruce ML, Sirey JA (2009). Caregiving tasks and training interest of family caregivers of medically ill homebound older adults. *Journal of Aging Health,* 21(3):528–542.

Wimo A et al. (2003). The magnitude of dementia occurence in the world. *Alzheimer Disease and Associated Disorders,* 17:63–67.

Zagorsky JL (2004). Is obesity as dangerous to wealth as it is to your health? *Research on Aging,* 26:130–152.

Zatonski WA, McMichael AJ, Powles JW (1998). Ecological study of reasons for sharp decline in mortality from ischaemic heart disease in Poland since 1991. *BMJ,* 316:1047–1051.

Zentner A, Velasco-Garrido M, Busse R (2005). *Methoden der vergleichenden Bewertung pharmazeutischer Produkte.* Köln/Berlin, DIMI/TU Berlin (http://www.egms.de/en/journals/hta/2005-1/hta000009.shtml, accessed 25 August 2008).

Zwar N et al. (2006). *A systematic review of chronic disease management.* Sydney, Australian Primary Health Care Institute.

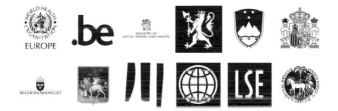

The European Observatory on Health Systems and Policies supports and promotes evidence-based health policy-making through comprehensive and rigorous analysis of health systems in Europe. It brings together a wide range of policy-makers, academics and practitioners to analyse trends in health reform, drawing on experience from across Europe to illuminate policy issues.

The European Observatory on Health Systems and Policies is a partnership between the World Health Organization Regional Office for Europe, the Governments of Belgium, Finland, Norway, Slovenia, Spain and Sweden, the Veneto Region of Italy, the European Investment Bank, the World Bank, the London School of Economics and Political Science and the London School of Hygiene & Tropical Medicine.

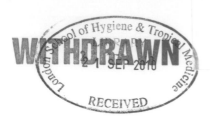

Tackling chronic disease in Europe